A Functional Medicine Monograph

GASTROINTESTINAL DYSREGULATION:

Connections to Chronic Disease

Leo Galland, MD
with Helen Lafferty, MB, MRCPI

IFM
THE INSTITUTE FOR FUNCTIONAL MEDICINE

A Nonprofit Educational Organization
www.functionalmedicine.org

Gastrointestinal Dysregulation: Connections to Chronic Disease
Leo Galland, MD, with Helen Lafferty, MB, MRCPI

4411 Pt. Fosdick Dr NW, Ste 305
P.O. Box 1697
Gig Harbor, WA 98335
800-228-0622
www.functionalmedicine.org

Disclaimer
This publication is intended only for use as an educational tool to broaden the knowledge and perspective of health practitioners. Nothing herein is intended to substitute for an individualized, thoughtful decision process by patients and providers. Clinically related material is not presented as a prescription for treatment, but rather as an indicator of the kind of information clinicians may want to consider in making treatment decisions for their patients. Neither the publisher, the authors, the editors, nor the reviewer assume any liability for any injury and/or damage to persons or property arising from the information to be found in this publication.

Project Team
Allison Templet, Project Manager and Editor
Sheila Quinn, Planning and Content Development
Gerry Mullin, MD, Technical Reviewer
Mary Smith, Cover Design
D. Kari Luraas, Interior Design and Layout
Lynn Siefken, Illustrator

ISBN-10: 0-9773713-5-2
ISBN-13: 978-0-9773713-5-8

Contents

Continuing Medical Education General Information v

Preface ix

Chapter 1 The Scope of the Problem: Prevalence of Gut-Associated Inflammation and its Impact on Systemic Disease 1

Introduction 1
Gluten Sensitivity, Gastrointestinal Inflammation, and Systemic Disease 2
Helicobacter pylori, Gastrointestinal Inflammation, and Systemic Disease 6
Inflammatory Bowel Disease, Gastrointestinal Inflammation, and Systemic Disease 9
Gastrointestinal Inflammation and the Spondyloarthritides 13
Gastrointestinal Inflammation and Cancer 15
Emerging Issues in Gastrointestinal Inflammation: Irritable Bowel Syndrome 16
Summary 19
References 19

Chapter 2 Flora, Intestinal Permeability, and Immune Response 25

Components and Functions of Gastrointestinal Defense 26
Gastrointestinal Dysfunction: Causes of Dysbiosis and Increased Permeability 32
Disease Manifestations of Dysbiosis, Permeability, and Immune Dysregulation 45
Summary 49
References 49

Chapter 3 Conventional Approaches to Treatment of Gastrointestinal and Systemic Diseases 57

Inflammatory Bowel Disease and Irritable Bowel Syndrome 57
Rheumatoid Arthritis and Fibromyalgia 61
Summary 64
References 64

Chapter 4 Antecedents, Triggers, and Mediators: A Functional Approach 67

Inflammatory Bowel Disease 69
Irritable Bowel Syndrome 74
Rheumatoid Arthritis 77
Fibromyalgia 81

Summary ... 85
References ... 85

Chapter 5 Clinical Applications: Applying Functional Medicine to Gut Dysregulation ... 93

Core Clinical Imbalances and the Functional Medicine Matrix Model ... 93
Case Reports ... 102
Concluding Remarks ... 107
References ... 107

Appendix The 4R Program ... 111

About the Authors ... 121

Continuing Medical Education General Information

Accreditation Statement

The Institute for Functional Medicine (IFM) is accredited by the Accreditation Council for Continuing Medical Education (ACCME) to provide continuing medical education (CME) for physicians.

Commercial Support

This CME activity is supported by educational grants from Doctor's Data Inc., Genova Diagnostics, InnoVision Health Media Inc., Metagenics, Inc., Metametrix Clinical Laboratory, Nordic Naturals, Inc., SpectraCell Laboratories, Inc., Thorne Research, Inc., TID*health*, Vital Nutrients, Vitamin Research Products, and Xymogen.

Continuing Education Credit Designations

For MDs and DOs, IFM designates this educational activity for a maximum of 6 *AMA PRA Category 1 credit(s)™*. Physicians should only claim credit commensurate with the extent of their participation in the activity.

Release date: May 22, 2008
Expiration date: May 22, 2011
Medium: Monograph

Method of Participation

To obtain CME credit for your participation in this activity:

1. Please read this monograph.
2. Complete the online evaluation, which will be sent to you via e-mail after purchase of the monograph; if you have any questions about accessing or completing the evaluation, contact IFM Client Services by e-mailing client_services@fxmed.com or calling 800-228-0622.

Statement of Need

Gap analyses and needs assessments conducted by IFM demonstrate an urgency for education and new approaches in treating complex, chronic disease. Additionally, increasing evidence demonstrates that imbalances in gastrointestinal immune responses, permeability, and microflora contribute to the epidemic of chronic disease. While disease in the gastrointestinal tract itself may be easily recognizable, medical practitioners trained in an organ-system model may not recognize how inflammation that begins in the gut may manifest in signs, symptoms, and dysfunctions throughout the body. In an era of high stress, poor diet, environmental contamination, and heavy pharmaceutical use, patients are particularly vulnerable to impairments in gut function and thus to debilitating illness.

Learning Objectives

- Evaluate the evidence in order to connect gut dysregulation to diseases outside the gastrointestinal tract, including type 1 diabetes, atopic dermatitis, spondyloarthritis, and ischemic heart disease.
- Analyze environmental factors leading to gastrointestinal permeability, inflammation, and dysbiosis, as well as the local and systemic diseases that can result.
- Recognize antecedents, triggers, and mediators in patients presenting with inflammatory bowel disease, irritable bowel syndrome, fibromyalgia, and rheumatoid arthritis.
- Evaluate gut function and address patient environment and lifestyle issues as part of the diagnosis and treatment of chronic disease.

Purpose Statement

The purpose of this monograph is to improve understanding of the complex interconnections between gut immune responses, inflammation, and both local and systemic disease in order to reduce suffering, better control costs, and improve outcomes of patients with chronic disease.

Who Should Participate?

Any specialist who cares for patients with chronic health problems, including primary care and specialist physicians.

Objectivity and Independence

It is the policy of IFM that all CME activities sponsored by IFM shall provide independent, balanced, objective, and scientifically rigorous presentations that are free of commercial bias. In accordance with ACCME Essential Areas and policies, IFM is totally responsible for all decisions on key components of activity development, including the development of activity goals and objectives, promotional material, content, faculty selection and approval, activity evaluation, and maintenance of physicians' credits.

Policy on Disclosure

As a sponsor accredited by ACCME, it is the policy of IFM to require all planners, authors, and editors to disclose (1) the existence of any relevant financial relationships with the supporters of this activity or manufacturer(s) of any commercial product(s) or services(s) that are discussed in their presentation, and (2) references in their presentations to unlabeled or unapproved use of drugs or devices. Disclosures are provided below.

Author Disclosure Statements

Leo Galland, MD, PC, is the president of Applied Nutrition, Inc., and he has indicated he receives an honorarium/salary from Allergy Research Group.

Helen Lafferty, MB, MRCPI, has indicated she has no financial relationships with any relevant commercial supporter or with the manufacturer of any commercial product or provider of any commercial service discussed in his presentation

Content Planner Disclosure Statements

David Jones, MD, is President and Director of Medical Education of the Institute for Functional Medicine.

Dan Lukaczer, ND, is Associate Director of Medical Education of the Institute for Functional Medicine.

Sheila Quinn has indicated she has no financial relationships with any relevant commercial supporter or with the manufacturer of any commercial product or provider of any commercial service relevant to this activity.

Allison Templet is project editor and coordinator at the Institute for Functional Medicine.

Preface

The Institute for Functional Medicine (IFM) is proud to present this remarkable monograph exploring the interconnections among gastrointestinal immune dysregulation, inflammation, and systemic pathology in chronic disease—an outstanding example of systems biology at work. IFM was most fortunate to secure Leo Galland, MD, as the lead author. A world-renowned physician and author, Dr. Galland developed the model of antecedents, triggers, and mediators of disease (now incorporated into the functional medicine paradigm), for which he received the Linus Pauling Award from IFM in 2000. He is a gifted writer and clinician, with a rare ability to articulate and clarify complex concepts. We are very grateful for his profound commitment to this work.

The gastrointestinal tract is our most intimate connection with the external world, providing both nourishment and protection and ceaselessly working to differentiate friend from foe in myriad ways. Although the gut has been viewed for centuries as one of the most important elements in health and disease, we are particularly vulnerable—in this era of high stress, poor diet, environmental contamination, and heavy pharmaceutical use—to impairments in gut function, thus creating vulnerability to a variety of chronic diseases. It is easy to overlook the many systemic ramifications of inflammation in the gut; most medical practitioners were trained in an organ-system model that doesn't emphasize searching for these underlying interconnections. This monograph offers a powerful rationale for including gut function in every comprehensive assessment of chronic disease and for treating gut dysfunction and its underlying causes wherever indicated. It presents the Functional Medicine Matrix Model as a tool for integrating gut assessment and treatment into clinical practice.

Using conditions that exemplify particularly well the connections between inflammatory processes in the gastrointestinal tract and a wide range of dysfunctions and diseases, this monograph explores the epidemiology (prevalence and costs of these conditions are very high), mechanisms (e.g., gluten sensitivity, *Helicobacter pylori* infection, use of nonsteroidal anti-inflammatory drugs), conventional management, and functional medicine approaches to irritable bowel syndrome, inflammatory bowel disease, rheumatoid arthritis, and fibromyalgia, among others. The use of antecedents, triggers, and mediators—as part of the Functional Medicine Matrix Model—is integrated into the discussion.

The value of eliciting and analyzing information about patient genetics, environment, and lifestyle choices—all important elements in the prevalence of most chronic gut conditions—is compellingly presented. The critical role of disturbances in gastrointestinal flora (dysbiosis) and intestinal permeability in disease pathogenesis (both local and systemic) is thoroughly explored. Dr. Galland clearly demonstrates how the failure to remediate imbalances in gut flora and intestinal permeability, as well as to address patient environment and lifestyle issues, contributes to the chronicity of many debilitating conditions. The cases presented at the end of the monograph integrate these concepts into clinical practice and demonstrate the critical thinking skills required of a functional medicine practitioner.

We hope this monograph serves as a wake-up call for all clinicians, challenging us to serve our patients with far greater efficacy through an improved understanding of the many complex interconnections between gut dysregulation, inflammation, and both local and system disease. We can reduce suffering, better control costs, and fundamentally alter the patient's disease trajectory back toward health if we fully embrace the concepts presented herein.

We gratefully acknowledge the skill with which Alex Vasquez, DC, ND, OMSII, presented the Functional Medicine Matrix Model in his monograph on musculoskeletal pain. Using some of that material in this monograph has enabled IFM to present the information in a clear and consistent way across both publications.

Dr. Galland's support team included medical writer Helen Lafferty, MB, MRCPI, technical reviewer Gerald Mullin, MD, project manager and editor Allison Templet, generous consultation and advice in the early months from Patrick Hanaway, MD, and early help in planning and content development from Sheila Quinn. Many thanks to all of them!

David S. Jones, MD
President and Director of Medical Education
The Institute for Functional Medicine

Chapter 1

The Scope of the Problem: Prevalence of Gut-Associated Inflammation and its Impact on Systemic Disease

Introduction

The gastrointestinal tract is essentially an external space enclosed within the body, an internalized interface between the human host and the outside world that is in constant contact with potential nutrients, as well as a vast array of drugs, microbes, toxins, and other foreign antigens. The total mucosal surface area of the adult gastrointestinal tract is over 200-fold greater than the surface area of the skin, making it the body's largest surface area that interacts with the environment.[1] The gastrointestinal tract not only assimilates vital nutrients and expels waste but also samples antigens and initiates and modifies immune responses; it is "the site where the divergent needs of nutrient absorption and host defense collide."[2] Disruptions of immune regulatory processes in the gastrointestinal tract have profound effects on inflammatory processes and responses throughout the body, giving them a role in the initiation and continuation of many seemingly disparate signs and symptoms, syndromes, and diseases that clinicians encounter on a daily basis.

While it is easy to imagine that immune dysregulation initiated at the level of the gastrointestinal tract results in dysfunction and disease in the tract itself, the far-reaching effects of inflammation in the gut may be less easily appreciated. In this monograph, we will address the connections between inflammatory processes occurring in the gastrointestinal tract and a wide range of dysfunctions and diseases as seemingly unrelated to the gut as type 1 diabetes, atopic dermatitis, spondyloarthritis, and ischemic heart disease. The overarching theme of this monograph is that a high degree of awareness of the connection between gut immune dysregulation, uncontrolled inflammation, and systemic pathology is necessary when treating patients with chronic disease.

In Chapter 1, we will examine the diversity of systemic dysfunction associated with gut immune dysregulation and inflammation. We will first examine gluten sensitivity, using it as a model of the way in which gut inflammation (induced in this case by food antigens) can result in a wide array of signs, symptoms, and dysfunctions throughout the body. Next we will discuss how gut inflammation induced by the microbe *Helicobacter pylori* also casts a wide arc of effects and induces dysfunction in remote parts of the body. We will then discuss the associations between gut inflammation and systemic disease in inflammatory bowel disease, as well as the role of gut inflammation in the pathogenesis of spondyloarthritis and cancer. And we will finish the chapter with a brief discussion of the emerging role of gut inflammation in irritable bowel syndrome.

In Chapter 2, we will discuss concepts important to an understanding of gut inflammation and its role in systemic disease. These concepts include the immunology of the gastrointestinal tract and the role of microbes residing there, the gastrointestinal flora. We will discuss environmental factors that can lead to gut immune dysregulation and to dysbiosis, a harmful state in which the composition of gut flora is altered. The balance of gut flora—commensal microbes vs. dysbiosis—is a key determinant in the development of a competent intestinal and systemic immune system.

In Chapter 3, we will review conventional approaches to four conditions (irritable bowel syndrome, inflammatory bowel disease, fibromyalgia, rheumatoid arthritis) in which gut inflammation and dysbiosis are postulated to play a part, then in Chapter 4, we will introduce the concepts of antecedents, triggers, and mediators of disease as a different way to approach patients with these difficult conditions. Finally, we will present a functional medicine approach to evaluation and treatment of these conditions, along with relevant case studies.

Gluten Sensitivity, Gastrointestinal Inflammation, and Systemic Disease

The association between inflammation in the gastrointestinal tract and systemic disease is nowhere more apparent than in the case of gluten sensitivity. Celiac disease was historically considered to be a purely gastrointestinal disease, a rare childhood malabsorption syndrome triggered by the ingestion of gluten-containing grains including wheat, barley, and rye.[3-5] The disease was associated with frank gastrointestinal symptoms (diarrhea, abdominal pain, weight loss, bloating) and failure to thrive; the finding of positive antigliadin antibody in the blood and villous atrophy on a small bowel biopsy, along with symptomatic and histological improvement on a gluten-free diet and relapse with reintroduction of gluten to the diet, confirmed the diagnosis.[3, 6] Currently, celiac disease (or, more broadly, gluten sensitivity) is considered to be a *common, systemic, T-cell-mediated autoimmune disease* of genetically susceptible individuals in whom exposure to gluten triggers an inflammatory response in the small intestine, leading to destruction of the villous structure.

Celiac disease is associated with a wide variety of extraintestinal manifestations that go far beyond the classic picture of malabsorption.[5, 7-10] Indeed, Fasano[11] noted that the disease can manifest with symptoms "potentially affecting any organ or body system." The number of extraintestinal diseases and dysfunctions associated with celiac disease is so great, and the extent of gastrointestinal symptomatology often so small, that celiac disease has been called "the great modern-day imposter,"[4] a "clinical chameleon."[12] Hadjivassiliou et al reported that this evidence of the diverse manifestations of celiac disease has necessitated "a re-evaluation of the belief that gluten sensitivity is solely a disease of the gut."[5]

According to the diagnostic criteria proposed by Marsh,[6] celiac disease should be diagnosed only when total villous atrophy along with crypt hyperplasia is seen on small bowel histology. However, it is now clear that many patients with gluten sensitivity have only minor histological changes in the small bowel.[13-15] Furthermore, even antibody tests can sometimes be negative in patients with early celiac disease.[16] These findings have prompted some authors to suggest that the diagnostic criteria should be widened[13] or even that the term *gluten sensitivity* should replace *celiac disease* as a more appropriate name for the disease.[5] A National Institutes of Health (NIH) consensus statement, released in 2004, recognized these difficulties and pointed out that "there is no one test that can definitively diagnose or exclude celiac disease in every individual," that "there is a continuum of laboratory and histopathologic results," and that "the combination of clinical and laboratory features may result in a diagnosis of celiac disease."[17] These statements suggest that the hard and fast criteria for diagnosing celiac disease based on the presence of villous atrophy are being replaced by a more expansive set of diagnostic criteria that take into account histological changes of varying degree, serological markers of gluten sensitivity, and response to a gluten-free diet. We prefer the term gluten sensitivity here, as it more accurately describes the wide range of histological changes and disease manifestations associated with sensitivity to gluten.

The changing picture of celiac disease makes its true prevalence difficult to ascertain. The classic picture of weight loss, diarrhea, steatorrhea, and anemia is still occasionally seen; estimates of the prevalence of celiac disease diagnosed on the basis of clinical presentation with classic symptoms range from 0.05% to 0.27%.[8] In several studies of general populations using antibody screening tests with small bowel biopsy for definitive diagnosis, the prevalence in both children and adults was found to be about 1%.[4, 8, 18-22] The prevalence in at-risk populations (including relatives of people with celiac disease, patients with symptoms associated with celiac disease such as diarrhea or abdominal pain, and patients with disorders associated with celiac disease such as diabetes mellitus, Down syndrome, arthritis, osteoporosis, and short stature) is much higher, ranging from 1.47% to 4.55% in a study by Fasano et al.[22]

These figures suggest that the ratio of clinically diagnosed to undetected cases is about 1 to 8. This discrepancy means that for every patient with clinically obvious signs of celiac disease seen in medical practice, there will be 7 or 8 more patients with celiac disease who present with atypical symptoms. This phenomenon has become known as the "celiac iceberg,"[7, 8] and in practice it means that, despite the fact that celiac disease is so prevalent and detectable that it meets the World Health Organization (WHO) criteria for mass screening,[11] patients with celiac disease often remain undiagnosed for many years. In a Canadian study of 2681 adults with biopsy-proven celiac disease, the mean delay in diagnosis was 11.7 years. Diagnoses made prior to celiac disease included anemia (40%), stress (31%), and irritable bowel syndrome (29%); 27% of respondents had consulted 3 or more doctors about their symptoms prior to diagnosis.[23] In a similar study in the United States, symptoms had been present for a mean of 11 years before diagnosis; only 52% of patients considered diagnosis prompt, and 31% of patients had consulted 2 or more gastroenterologists prior to eventual diagnosis.[24] Clearly, then, the fact that celiac disease is a common disease with "protean manifestations"[17] has not translated into sufficient awareness among practitioners.

The immunologic and inflammatory nature of celiac disease has been extensively studied. Briefly, the development of celiac disease is believed to require 4 components: gluten, genetic susceptibility (in the form of major histocompatibility complex locus HLA-DQ), T cells, and the endogenous enzyme tissue transglutaminase.[2, 7, 9, 25] In genetically susceptible individuals, gluten peptides, which are deamidated by tissue transglutaminase (an enzyme found in epithelial cells in the small intestine), bind to antigen-presenting cells in the lamina propria. The deamidated peptides stimulate the adaptive immune system to produce antibodies to gliadin, as well as to tissue transglutaminase, which acts as the autoantigen in celiac disease.[2, 3, 5, 7, 9, 25] In addition to this adaptive T-cell-mediated response, it appears that a nonantigenic portion of gluten also acts to stimulate a nonspecific immediate response of the innate immune system, driven by interleukin-15, which is responsible for damage to the mucosa and which predates and facilitates T-cell recognition of antigenic gliadin peptides.[26] Some authors have also proposed a primary role for intestinal hyperpermeability, induced by gliadin, in the pathogenesis of the disease.[7] And research suggests possible roles for environmental triggers such as *Candida albicans*,[10] bacteria,[27] or viruses[28] in initiating immune responses to gliadin. Cross-reactivity of transglutaminase and gliadin antibodies with a variety of antigens, including antigens in skin[29] and nerve[30] systems, appears to play a role in the pathogenesis of many of the diverse systemic diseases associated with gluten intolerance.

For the purposes of emphasizing the effect of inflammation initiated in the gut on multiple body systems, as well as the diverse ways in which gastrointestinal inflammatory diseases can manifest themselves, we will concentrate here on the extraintestinal manifestations of celiac disease. The list of systemic disorders associated with celiac disease is enormous, and a full review of these conditions is beyond the scope of this monograph. Celiac disease has been noted to have hematologic,[31] rheumatologic,[32] bone,[33] neurological,[34] endocrine,[35, 36] hepatic,[37] dental,[38] and cutaneous[29, 39] presentations and associations. In addition, it has been found to be associated with many organ-specific[40, 41] and non-organ-specific autoimmune diseases[7] and an increased incidence of various malignant conditions including carcinoma of the oropharynx, esophagus, and jejunum and intestinal lymphoma.[42] Associations of uncertain etiology include dental enamel defects.[38, 43] Table 1.1 provides a list of clinical features, conditions, and complications associated with celiac disease.

Certain disorders seen in celiac patients are due to malabsorption of nutrients secondary to small bowel mucosal damage.[25] Patients may present with microcytic anemia secondary to iron deficiency or with macrocytic anemia secondary to malabsorption of folate and vitamin B12. Symptoms associated with these deficiencies include fatigue and neuropsychiatric disorders such as peripheral neuropathy, ataxia, paraesthesia, and memory loss.[45] Deficiencies of fat-soluble vitamins A, D, K, and E may also occur (more commonly in patients with classic celiac disease[25]), with the associated symptoms and signs (night blindness, conjunctival dryness, and keratomalacia in vitamin A deficiency; osteomalacia with muscle weakness and pain in vitamin D deficiency; excessive bleeding in vitamin K deficiency; and hemolytic anemia, gait disturbances, and neuropathy in vitamin E deficiency).[25]

Table 1.1—Clinical Presentations of Celiac Disease[3]

Common Features	Less Common Features	Associated Conditions	Complications
Adults • Iron-deficiency anemia • Diarrhea **Children** • Diarrhea • Failure to thrive • Abdominal distention	**General** • Short stature • Delayed puberty **Gastrointestinal** • Recurrent aphthous stomatitis • Recurrent abdominal pain • Steatorrhea **Extraintestinal** • Folate-deficiency anemia • Osteopenia or osteoporosis • Dental-enamel hypoplasia • Vitamin K deficiency • Hypertransaminasemia • Thrombocytosis (hyposplenism) • Arthralgia or arthropathy • Polyneuropathy • Ataxia • Epilepsy (with or without cerebral calcification) • Infertility • Recurrent abortions • Anxiety and depression • Follicular keratosis • Alopecia	**Definite associations** • Dermatitis herpetiformis • IgA deficiency • Type 1 diabetes • Autoimmune thyroid disease • Sjögren's syndrome • Microscopic colitis • Rheumatoid arthritis • Down syndrome • IgA nephropathy **Possible associations** • Congenital heart disease • Recurrent pericarditis • Sarcoidosis • Cystic fibrosis • Fibrosing alveolitis • Lung cavities • Pulmonary hemosiderosis • Inflammatory bowel disease • Autoimmune hepatitis • Primary biliary cirrhosis • Addison's disease • Systemic lupus erythematosus • Vasculitis • Polymyositis • Myasthenia gravis • Schizophrenia	• Refractory sprue • Enteropathy-associated T-cell lymphoma • Carcinoma of the oropharynx, esophagus, and small bowel • Ulcerative jejunoileitis • Collagenous sprue

Several studies have examined the association between celiac disease and organ-specific autoimmune disorders, which can serve as a model for other gut-associated relationships. Data on the association between celiac disease and type 1 diabetes are plentiful.[40, 41, 46, 47] In a large population-based study in Sweden, patients with diagnosed celiac disease were found on screening to have a significantly increased risk (2- to 3-fold) of subsequent type 1 diabetes.[41] (It is worth noting here that since the authors assessed only patients with diagnosed celiac disease, some of whom had been diagnosed as far back as 1964, they may have underestimated the true magnitude of the association since they almost certainly omitted some number of patients with latent or silent celiac disease.) In a 6-year prospective longitudinal study of patients with type 1 diabetes, there was a significantly increased risk of developing celiac disease over the 6-year period, although the rate of diagnosis fell off after 4 years.[47] However, the authors noted that in 60% of the patients, celiac disease was already present at the time of diagnosis of diabetes, suggesting that celiac disease predated the development of diabetes in these patients. Because of the often latent and undiagnosed nature of celiac disease and the lack of screening, we do not know for certain whether celiac disease typically predates the onset of diabetes, so the temporal relationship is unclear. Yet the association between celiac disease and type 1 diabetes is not in doubt, and *screening for celiac disease is recommended in all patients with type 1 diabetes*.[40, 47, 48] Furthermore, the role of gluten sensitivity in the pathogenesis of type 1 diabetes has been suggested by studies finding that early introduction of gluten to children at high risk for type 1 diabetes produces islet cell autoantibodies[49] and that some children with celiac disease but without diabetes have high levels of islet cell antibodies that disappear on a gluten-free diet.[50]

Several studies have found an association between celiac disease and autoimmune thyroid disorders.[35, 36, 51-53] In one study, the prevalence of celiac disease in Graves' disease patients was found on antibody screening to be 4.5%, compared with 0.9% in the general population, with celiac disease being undiagnosed in all patients prior to the study.[53] In another screening study, the prevalence of celiac disease (again undiagnosed in all cases prior to the study) was significantly higher in patients with Graves' disease and Hashimoto's thyroiditis than in controls. In this study, the presence of other autoimmune diseases was also significantly higher in the celiac group than in controls.[51]

In a study that looked at the association from the other direction, newly diagnosed celiac patients were screened for the presence of thyroid disorders. (Interestingly, in this study, the clinical pattern of celiac disease was atypical in 40% of patients and completely silent in a further 16%.[35]) Thyroid disease, including both autoimmune thyroid disease with euthyroidism and autoimmune hypothyroidism, was 3-fold higher in celiac patients than in controls, and the prevalence of thyroid antibody positivity in euthyroid subjects was 4-fold higher in celiac patients than in controls. In several of the patients, normalization of thyroid function, in both autoimmune and non-autoimmune types, was achieved by adherence to a gluten-free diet.[35] In a separate study of the prevalence of thyroid disease in patients with an established diagnosis of celiac disease, 43% had abnormalities of thyroid function (subclinical or clinical hypothyroidism in all but 1 patient), and almost 50% had positivity for thyroid antibodies.[54] Another study found an association between the major depressive disorder sometimes seen in celiac patients and the presence of thyroid antibodies.[36]

One of the most well-studied neurological disorders associated with celiac disease is cerebellar ataxia.[34] In a 2005 review[34] of studies examining the neurological manifestations of celiac disease, the prevalence of biopsy-proven celiac disease was found to range from 1.9% to 16% of patients with cerebellar ataxia of unknown cause, and the prevalence of positive antigliadin antibodies in these patients ranged from 0% to 41%. Some reports suggested that a gluten-free diet improves ataxic symptoms.[55] Other neurological abnormalities noted to occur in association with celiac disease include epilepsy, dementia, depression, peripheral neuropathy, migraine, encephalopathy, chorea, brain stem dysfunction, myelopathy, mononeuritis multiplex, and Guillain-Barré-like syndrome.[34] Down syndrome has also been noted to have an association with celiac disease.[56] In terms of etiology, several studies suggested that cross-reactivity between gluten antibodies and neuronal antigens are implicated in the pathogenesis of neurological diseases associated with celiac disease, suggesting an autoimmune pathogenesis.[30, 57]

Celiac disease has been associated with several other diseases thought to be autoimmune in nature. For example, gluten sensitivity is associated with Sjögren's syndrome, a disease considered to be the second most common rheumatic autoimmune disease, with a prevalence in the United States of between 2 million and 4 million people.[58] Several studies have assessed celiac disease in Sjögren's syndrome patients, finding a prevalence that ranges from 4.5% to 14.7%.[59-61] (Interestingly, 2 review articles[58, 62] on the clinical manifestations of Sjögren's syndrome failed to mention the association with celiac disease, prompting, in one case, a letter to the journal to point out the omission.[63]) There are also several cutaneous manifestations of celiac disease,[29] the most well-known of which is dermatitis herpetiformis, an immune-mediated, probably autoimmune, disease of the skin that is considered to be a dermatologic variant of celiac disease; it is characterized by granular IgA deposits in the dermal papillae and responds to treatment with gluten-free diet. The autoantigen is considered to be epidermal transglutaminase.[64] (A 2004 article noted that subsequent to the discovery that dermatitis herpetiformis was a dermatologic manifestation of celiac disease in the late 1960s, the response "should have been the realization of the sys-

Clinical Pearl:

In my personal clinical experience,[i] every patient I have seen with Sjögren's syndrome has experienced benefit from a gluten-free diet. Benefits have included healing of skin ulcers and relief of cognitive dysfunction caused by Sjögren-associated vasculitis.

[i] First-person singular usage in the text identifies the monograph's lead author.

temic nature of the immune response in the pathogenesis of gluten sensitivity. Yet, clinicians and scientists failed to capitalize on this important observation and celiac disease was considered, almost exclusively, a disease of the gut for years to come, with abnormalities always attributed to malabsorption, particularly of vitamins."[5]) Alopecia areata [65] and psoriasis[66-69] are also autoimmune skin disorders associated with celiac disease. Although results are conflicting, there are at least some reports on alopecia areata in which hair growth resumed with a gluten-free diet.[70-72]

Other conditions thought to have an inflammatory or autoimmune component that are also associated with celiac disease include migraine,[73, 74] depression,[34, 36, 75] arthritis,[3, 4, 32, 76] and malignancies (in particular, epithelial tumors of the digestive tract and lymphomas of both B and T cell types).[42, 77-79] The possibility of malignancy in unrecognized celiac disease is a particular cause for concern, since an increased overall cancer mortality has been reported in celiac patients.[42] A recent review[80] of data concerning the protective effect of a gluten-free diet on the development of malignancy suggested that strict adherence to a such a diet appears to reduce overall relative risk for cancer over time.

There is an ongoing debate about the wisdom of screening the population at large for celiac disease.[11, 81] Larger studies would help to further elucidate the natural history of undetected gluten sensitivity and celiac disease.[8] In clinical practice, however, there should be a high level of awareness of gluten sensitivity and the myriad ways in which it can present. Despite the fact that gut inflammation is the primary lesion in gluten sensitivity and celiac disease, we have shown in this section that patients with gluten intolerance (or celiac disease) may have no gastrointestinal symptoms, may have symptoms related to other body systems, or may have no specific organ-related symptoms at all. Indeed, in one study, fatigue was the presenting symptom in 82% of celiac patients.[82]

Interestingly, it is difficult to find information about the burdens and costs associated with celiac disease in the medical literature, perhaps reflecting the fact that the disease was previously thought to be so rare. We note, with dismay, that the "Burden of Gastrointestinal Diseases" report issued in 2001 by the American Gastroenterological Association includes no information on celiac disease.[83] It is likely, however, that the costs of appropriate treatment for celiac disease and its associated disorders, both in terms of patient burden and medical care, are substantial, given the many manifestations that arise and the various organ systems that can be affected. However, when we consider the additional and unnecessary costs incurred through incorrect or long-delayed diagnosis, leading to inappropriate treatment, we can perceive a far greater cost burden than simply treating the appropriately diagnosed disease.

Several important conclusions can be drawn from the information presented above:

- Gluten sensitivity is a common condition in which the primary pathology involves inflammation in the gastrointestinal tract.
- The gut inflammation associated with gluten sensitivity has effects that can reach many different organ systems.
- Gluten sensitivity may present with a vast array of signs and symptoms; gastrointestinal symptoms may be minimal or absent.
- Autoimmune disease related to gluten sensitivity and celiac disease is common.
- Missed or delayed diagnosis of gluten sensitivity is extremely common.
- A gluten-free diet results in resolution of symptoms, while continued exposure to gluten accelerates disease progression.

Helicobacter pylori, Gastrointestinal Inflammation, and Systemic Disease

H. pylori is the most common chronic bacterial infection affecting humans[84] and is present in approximately half of the world's population.[85] First cultured in 1984, *H. pylori* is a gram-negative spiral bacterium with a particular affinity for gastric mucosa. Though only a small proportion of infected individuals experience clinical illness, this bacterium is now known to be causally implicated in several gastrointestinal diseases, including peptic ulcer disease,[84, 86] gastric cancer,[87-89] and gastric lymphoma.[88, 90]

A recent review[91] summarized the epidemiological features of *H. pylori*: The prevalence of *H. pylori* is far higher in developing countries (the rate of infection at age 60 approaches 100% in India). Density of living conditions seems to be a significant risk factor for acquisition of *H. pylori*, and the prevalence of infection in developed countries is inversely related to socioeconomic status. Gastro-oral and fecal-oral are the most common routes of transmission, occurring mainly within families. Infection is usually acquired in childhood, though there is typically a long period of latency, with disease manifestations not appearing until adulthood. The prevalence appears to be decreasing, probably due to changes in standards of living, changes in medical practice leading to greater use of antimicrobials, and spontaneous loss of infection.[91]

Based on the well-documented association between the chronic gastritis induced by *H. pylori* and both peptic ulcer disease[84, 86] and gastric malignancy,[87-90] the bacterium has come to be recognized over the past 2 decades as a major public health problem worldwide. In 1994, the International Agency for Research on Cancer classified the bacterium as carcinogenic.[92] Furthermore, resistance to antimicrobial therapy used to eliminate pathogens such as *H. pylori* is emerging as a major public health problem.[86] Here, we concentrate on the associations between *H. pylori* and a number of extra-gastric diseases that may be less well recognized in clinical practice.

Several authors have discussed the immunopathology of *H. pylori* infection, either in the context of specific diseases[93-97] or as general reviews.[93, 98-100] Briefly, this opportunistic bacterium, once it gains entry into the stomach, induces a sustained immune response. Both cellular and humoral responses occur subsequent to the attachment of *H. pylori* to host cells, and disruption of intestinal permeability also accompanies the initial immunologic response.[98-100] The inflammation induced in the stomach progresses through superficial gastritis, chronic atrophic gastritis, intestinal metaplasia, and dysplasia to eventual carcinoma in some patients.[101] Molecular mimicry between *H. pylori* antigens and antigens in other parts of the body, including vascular smooth muscle cells[95] or other endothelial cells,[93] sympathetic neurons,[97] and platelets,[96, 99] appears to be important in the development of systemic autoimmune disease. Most people infected with *H. pylori* have asymptomatic gastritis, with gastric cancer occurring in approximately 1% of affected individuals.[100] (For more information on the role of gastrointestinal inflammation in cancer pathogenesis, see *Gastrointestinal Inflammation and Cancer* below.)

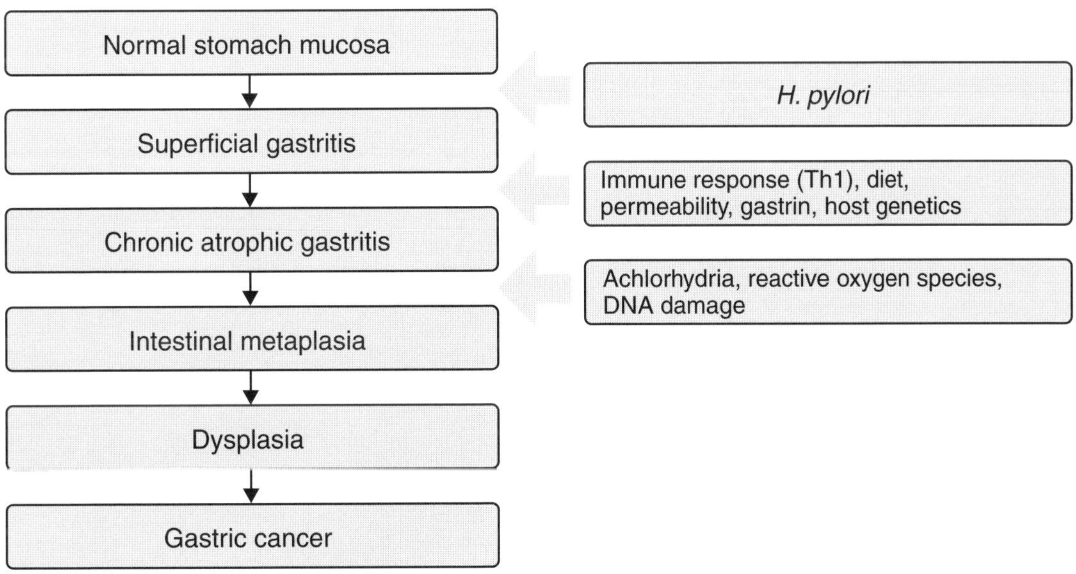

Figure 1.1—*H. pylori* in Cancer Pathogenesis

Source: Kusters JG, van Vliet AHM, Kuipers EJ. Pathogenesis of *Helicobacter pylori* infection. *Clin Microbiol Rev*. 2006;19:449-490.

As mentioned earlier, gut inflammation induced by *H. pylori* induces dysfunction in remote parts of the body, and several disease associations are discussed below. (For a discussion of possible mechanisms by which microbes induce disease, see Chapter 2, *Flora, Intestinal Permeability, and Immune Response.*)

Ischemic heart disease and cerebrovascular disease — The substantial research on this association has been documented in a recent review by Franceschi and Gasbarrini,[102] who examined in particular the possible role of chronic infection in the development of atherosclerotic plaques and vessel-wall injury. A recent meta-analysis[85] of several studies, both retrospective and prospective, found a small but significant association between virulent (CagA-positive) strains of *H. pylori* and both ischemic heart disease and cerebrovascular disease. The researchers who performed the meta-analysis pointed out that since these virulent strains of *H. pylori* are found in 30% of the population worldwide, even small associations may have important epidemiological consequences. Of course, at the level of the individual patient, eradicating any risk factor for ischemic heart disease and stroke is always important. The finding of cross-reactivity between anti-CagA antibodies and vascular wall antigens by Franceschi et al,[95] as well as the finding of *H. pylori* DNA in atherosclerotic plaques associated with features of inflammatory cell response,[103] lends further credence to the idea that the bacterium is causally implicated in vascular disease.

Idiopathic thrombocytopenic purpura — *H. pylori* appears to be associated with this autoimmune disease characterized by autoantibody-mediated destruction of platelets.[104] Several studies have demonstrated that eradication of *H. pylori* in patients with idiopathic thrombocytopenic purpura, particularly children, results in increases in platelet counts in a percentage of these patients, especially if the disease is of short duration.[105-108] In a recent randomized controlled trial, adults with chronic idiopathic thrombocytopenic purpura and *H. pylori* colonization of the stomach (confirmed by culture of gastric biopsy specimens) were randomized to receive either eradication treatment or no treatment. A significant difference in platelet recovery was observed between the groups, with 46% of patients in the eradication group showing complete or partial response and no patients in the non-eradication group showing improvement.[109]

Iron-deficiency anemia — Several studies have shown that eradication of *H. pylori* corrects hemoglobin levels in patients, particularly children, with iron-deficiency anemia that is not attributable to causes such as intestinal loss, poor intake, or malabsorption.[94, 110-114] In one interesting study, *H. pylori*-positive patients treated with either iron plus antibiotics or with antibiotics alone showed significant increases in serum hemoglobin after 8 weeks, whereas patients treated only with iron showed persistence of anemia.[115] While the mechanisms by which *H. pylori* causes iron deficiency are uncertain, it has been suggested that the bacterium may sequester iron in the gastric antrum[94] or that low gastric acid concentration and ascorbic acid levels secondary to infection-induced gastritis may impair alimentary iron absorption.[116]

Idiopathic anterior uveitis — In a study published in 2005, the authors found evidence of *H. pylori* infection in 6 of 15 patients with idiopathic anterior uveitis. In 3 of those patients, *H. pylori* antibodies were found in the aqueous humor,[117] suggesting an autoimmune process. The finding in another recent study of positive serology for *H. pylori* in 67% of uveitis patients, as well as in 80% of patients with both anterior uveitis and spondyloarthritis,[118] again suggests a link between the bacterium and uveitis (while also opening up the possibility of a link with spondyloarthritis—see *Gastrointestinal Inflammation and the Spondyloarthritides* below).

Parkinsonism — Yet another extraintestinal disorder in which *H. pylori* has been implicated is idiopathic parkinsonism.[97, 119] In a review of gut inflammation's role in the etiology and pathogenesis of parkinsonism, the authors noted that, until now, "the concept of a continually active, systemic disease, where any abnormal homeostatic state might be immunological, rather than metabolic, has been ignored."[97] Noting associations between idiopathic parkinsonism and peptic ulcer (reported before the discovery of *H. pylori*), as well as epidemiological similarities between *H. pylori* and idiopathic parkinsonism (including familial aggregation, linkage with sources of drinking water, and the fact that siblings of people with idiopathic parkinsonism have a 3-fold increase in odds of seropositivity for *H. pylori* antibodies), the authors concluded that "the candidacy of *Helicobacter pylori* infection as a trigger event or driving infection [for idiopathic parkinsonism] is relatively high."[97]

Autoimmune thyroid disease — A few studies in the late 1990s found an association between the prevalence of *H. pylori* gastric infection and the prevalence of autoimmune thyroid disease.[120, 121] And a more recent study, published in 2006, again found a significant association between positive serology for *H. pylori* and the presence of autoimmune thyroid disease.[122] Not all studies, however, have found this association.[123]

Mucosa-associated lymphoid tissue (MALT) lymphoma — These tumors usually arise in sites normally devoid of lymphoid tissue in the context of long-standing infection or autoimmune disease. The incidence of gastric MALT lymphomas is high in regions where *H. pylori* infection is endemic, and eradication of *H. pylori* leads to complete regression of lymphoma in the early stages of disease.[124]

Clinical Pearl:

Intriguingly, a published case reported on a patient in whom primary thyroid MALT lymphoma occurred in association with Hashimoto's thyroiditis; the patient also had gastric cancer associated with *H. pylori*. The thyroid tumor transiently decreased in size following a subtotal gastrectomy but disappeared completely after treatment to eradicate *H. pylori* infection.[125]

Other diseases that have been postulated to be associated with *H. pylori* include otitis media,[126] acne rosacea,[93, 127] open-angle glaucoma,[88] Sjögren's syndrome,[128] and food allergy.[129]

H. pylori is not the only microbe that infects the gastrointestinal tract and causes systemic disease. These other gut microbes include *Klebsiella pneumoniae* (implicated in the pathogenesis of spondyloarthritis[130, 131]), *Yersinia enterocolitica* (implicated in the pathogenesis of autoimmune thyroid disease[132] and reactive arthritis[133]), *Campylobacter jejuni* (implicated in the pathogenesis of reactive arthritis[133] and Guillain-Barré syndrome[134]), *Salmonella* (implicated in the pathogenesis of reactive arthritis[133]), *Escherichia coli* (implicated in the pathogenesis of hemolytic uremic syndrome[135]), and *C. albicans* (implicated in the pathogenesis of atopic dermatitis[136] and celiac disease[10]).

Even this brief discussion directs our attention to some critical points:

- *H. pylori* is a very common, and often silent, cause of gastrointestinal inflammation.
- The gut inflammation associated with *H. pylori* is implicated in the pathogenesis of several systemic diseases, and there appears to be an autoimmune connection. These diseases may present in ways that have no obvious relationship with gut pathology.
- Gut microbes other than *H. pylori* are also implicated in systemic disease.

Inflammatory Bowel Disease, Gastrointestinal Inflammation, and Systemic Disease

Ulcerative colitis and Crohn's disease are chronic, relapsing inflammatory diseases of the gastrointestinal tract. The clinical spectrum ranges from largely quiescent disease to life-threatening severe illness, and patients may require extensive medical and surgical interventions over many decades.[137, 138] Although ulcerative colitis and Crohn's disease are generally thought of as clinically distinct conditions, whether they are fundamentally distinct or part of a continuum of disease remains an unanswered question.[138, 139] While inflammation of the gastrointestinal tract is the hallmark of these diseases, extraintestinal manifestations are extremely common,[140, 141] and the immune and genetic mechanisms underlying these manifestations are being elucidated.[140, 141]

There are hundreds of articles describing the incidence and prevalence of Crohn's disease and ulcerative colitis in various parts of the world, including several comprehensive reviews.[142-144] Historically, the highest incidence and prevalence for both diseases have been reported in northern Europe, the United Kingdom, and the United States.[142] If the data for the areas with the highest prevalence are extrapolated, there may be more than 600,000 people with Crohn's disease and more than 690,000 people with ulcerative colitis in North America, for a combined total of over 1.3 million people.[142] Similarly, extrapolating figures across the European population suggests that as many as 2.2 million Europeans may be afflicted with inflammatory bowel disease.[144]

The current incidence rate of both Crohn's disease and ulcerative colitis is thought to be about 10 to 20 per 100,000 per year.[2] Since the early 1990s, the incidence and prevalence of both conditions have also been rising in parts of the developing world, including Eastern Europe, Asia, Africa, and Latin America.[143, 144] The incidence rates for both ulcerative colitis and Crohn's disease appear to have stabilized in areas with a previously high incidence, whereas incidence rates continue to rise in areas with a formerly low incidence.[144] Prevalence rates in the United States are lower in Hispanics and Asians than in whites and African-Americans, and both Crohn's disease and ulcerative colitis are more prevalent in Jewish people.[145] Crohn's disease appears to be slightly more common in females, whereas ulcerative colitis appears to be slightly more common in males.[142] Several studies have shown an increased incidence of pediatric inflammatory bowel disease (especially Crohn's disease) over the past decade.[143] A retrospective study of Australian children 16 and under who were diagnosed with Crohn's disease found that the incidence rate rose from 0.128 to 2.0 per 100,000 per year between 1971 and 2001.[146]

Variations in incidence among different populations, increased incidence (especially of Crohn's disease) in monozygotic twins, familial aggregation, and several animal studies all lend support to the notion that there is a genetic component involved in susceptibility to inflammatory bowel disease.[138] However, the dynamic nature of incidence rates of these diseases makes it clear that environmental factors are also important in their etiology.[138, 139, 145] Environmental factors appear to include the use of nonsteroidal anti-inflammatory drugs (which can lead to disease flares), early appendectomy (which is associated with a reduced incidence of ulcerative colitis), smoking (which protects against ulcerative colitis but increases the risk of Crohn's disease), changes in the composition of gastrointestinal flora,[138] and dietary changes related to "Westernization," although there is no clear consensus on the role of dietary factors in the epidemiology of inflammatory bowel disease.[144] The aggregate effect of these genetic predispositions and environmental triggers appears to be a sustained activation of gastrointestinal mucosal immune responses that is driven by the presence of normal gut flora.[138] Briefly, in Crohn's disease, there appears to be an excessive immune response to antigens of the normal gut flora, which results in an exaggerated T helper 1 (Th1) cell response with infiltration by macrophages.[2, 138, 147] In contrast, in ulcerative colitis, there is an excessive Th2 cell response to gut flora.[138, 147] Defects in barrier function also appear to be involved in the pathogenesis of both ulcerative colitis and Crohn's disease.[2, 138, 139] (For more information on alterations in gut flora and epithelial barrier function in inflammatory bowel disease, see *Disease Manifestations of Dysbiosis, Permeability, and Immune Dysregulation* in Chapter 2.)

Inflammatory bowel diseases have been noted to have "dismaying clinical manifestations,"[138] and it has been suggested that they should be considered systemic diseases rather than solely diseases of the gut.[148] Extraintestinal manifestations are common, with 20% to 40% of patients with inflammatory bowel disease displaying at least one[141]; extraintestinal manifestations may occur prior to, in conjunction with, or subsequent to active bowel disease.[140, 148, 149] The organs most commonly involved include the joints, bones, skin, eyes, and biliary tract, although almost all organ systems can be affected.[140, 141, 148] Extraintestinal manifestations are more common in Crohn's disease than ulcerative colitis.[149]

Clinical Pearl:

Although they are conventionally treated with the same medications, patients with Crohn's disease and ulcerative colitis tend to respond very differently to nutritional interventions. In my experience, patients with Crohn's often benefit from a high-protein, grain- and disaccharide-free diet, whereas patients with ulcerative colitis tend to benefit from a high-fiber, low-fat dietary pattern.

Joint complications are the most common extraintestinal manifestations of inflammatory bowel disease, affecting from 7% to 35% of patients.[141, 148, 149] One form of joint involvement is a peripheral, seronegative, nonerosive, transient, asymmetrical arthritis that occurs in 10% to 20% of patients and is similar to the reactive arthritis that occurs secondary to intestinal infection.[141, 149, 151] The second form of joint involvement in inflammatory bowel disease is an axial arthritis that may vary from asymptomatic sacroiliitis to inflammatory lower back pain to classic spondyloarthritis (see *Gastrointestinal Inflammation and the Spondyloarthritides* below); it occurs in 7% to 25% of patients with inflammatory bowel disease.[141, 148, 151] The most common bone manifestation is osteoporosis (thought

Table 1.2—Extraintestinal Manifestations of IBD[150]

Extraintestinal manifestations	Extraintestinal complications
Musculosceletal diseases	
Peripheral arthritis	Drug-induced osteoporosis and osteonecrosis
Ankylosing spondylitis	Bacterial infection of joints (fistulization, immunosuppression)
Isolated sacroiliitis	Septic arthritis
Metastatic Crohn's disease	
Mucocutaneous diseases	
Erythema nodosum	Anal fissures
Pyoderma gangraenosum	Fistulas
Aphthous stomatitis/oral ulceration	
Psoriasis?	Acrodermatitis enteropathica (zinc deficiency)
Epidermolysis bullosa acquisita?	Purpura (vitamin C and K deficiency)
Sweet syndrome?	Glossitis (vitamin B or zinc deficiency)
Erythema exsudativum multiforme?	Hair loss (protein deficiency)
	Brittle nail (protein deficiency)
	Perlèche (iron deficiency)
	Candidiasis (zinc deficiency, immunosuppression)
	Mucositis/stomatitis (methotrexate)
	Drug-induced rash, allergic exanthema
	Moon-face, acne, stretch marks, skin atrophy (steroid treatment)
Ocular diseases	
Anterior uveitis	Night blindness (vitamin A deficiency)
Conjunctivitis	Kerathopathy (vitamin A deficiency)
Iritis	Opportunistic infections (immunosuppressants)
Skleritis/episcleritis	
Hepatobiliary diseases	
Primary sclerosing cholangitis	Gallstones in Crohn's disease
Granulomatous Crohn's hepatitis	Fatty liver
Autoimmune chronic active hepatitis?	
Biliary cirrhosis?	
Pancreatic diseases	
Acute pancreatitis	Drug-induced pancreatitis (5-ASA, azathioprine)
Chronic pancreatitis, exocrine insuffciency	Biliary pancreatitis in Crohn's disease
	Duodenal involvement in Crohn's disease
Blood and vascular diseases	
Thrombembolic events	Anemia (iron, folate, vitamin B12 deficiency)
Autoimmune hemolytic anemia?	Thrombocytosis, leucocytosis
Thrombocytopenic purpura (Moschcowitz syndrome)?	Hypercoagulation: venous thrombosis, thrombembolism
Renal diseases	
Tubular proteinuria	Nephrolithiasis (oxalate stones, uric acid stones)
Glomerulonephritis?	Local affection involving the urethro-genital system
	Acute interstitial nephritis (drug-related SASP, 5-ASA)
Interstitial nephritis?	Drug-induced renal insufficiency (5-ASA, SASP, cyclosporine)
	Renal amyloidosis
Bronchopulmonary diseases	
Chronic bronchitis/bronchiolitis/bronchiectasis	Drug-induced hypersensitivity pneumonitis
Acute laryngotracheitis/ tracheal stenosis	Drug-related pulmonary fibrosis (methotrexate)
Bronchiolitis obliterans organizing pneumonia	Drug induced pleuritis
Pleuritis/ serositis	Opportunistic infections (immunosuppression)
Cardiac diseases	
Pericarditis	Drug-induced pericarditis (5-ASA)
Myocarditis?/perimyocarditis	
Neurological diseases	
Demyelinating diseases including multiple sclerosis	Peripheral neuropathy (vitamin B12 deficiency)
Optic neuritis, sensorial hearing loss	Drug-induced leucencephalopathia (natalizumab, infliximab)
Myasthenia gravis?	Drug-induced polyneuropathia (metronidazole)

to be due to an inflammatory process in the bone itself, as well as to malabsorption of vitamin D and calcium), which appears to be associated with a slightly higher risk of fracture.[141, 148, 152] Cutaneous manifestations include the granulomatous skin lesions seen in Crohn's disease patients (with histological features similar to those seen in the bowel) and the inflammatory lesions of erythema nodosum and pyoderma gangrenosum.[148, 149, 153] The most common hepatobiliary manifestation is primary sclerosing cholangitis, a condition characterized by inflammation and fibrosis of both intrahepatic and extrahepatic bile ducts.[141, 148, 149] In addition, there is an increased incidence of colon cancer observed in patients with long-standing inflammatory bowel disease (see *Gastrointestinal Inflammation and Cancer* below). [154, 155]

Although the pathogenesis of the extraintestinal manifestations of inflammatory bowel disease is still poorly understood, both genetic and immunologic mechanisms are thought to be implicated.[141] In terms of the immunologic pathogenesis of these manifestations, the dysregulated immune response to colonic bacteria that triggers the colonic injury also triggers T-cell- and cytokine-mediated inflammatory responses in extraintestinal organs. In addition, development of autoantibodies to antigens in various other organ systems may occur; cross-reactivity has been noted between colonic epithelial protein and epitopes found in eyes, chondrocytes, and biliary epithelium.[140, 141, 148] The finding that extraintestinal manifestations may occur even several years after the colon has been removed suggests that memory T cells may continue to circulate and thus can be reactivated after a stimulus.[148] In addition to these immune-mediated manifestations, other extraintestinal manifestations are caused by nutritional deficiencies and other metabolic disturbances secondary to the gastrointestinal dysfunction.[140]

Inflammatory bowel diseases are chronic, relapsing conditions associated with considerable morbidity. Because they usually occur during the economically productive years of a person's life, the burden borne both by patients and by society as a whole is enormous. Crohn's disease patients had more than 1 million physician office visits in the United States in 1998, almost 70,000 emergency room visits, and almost 85,000 inpatient hospital stays. Hospital inpatient treatment and drugs make up the bulk of direct costs of Crohn's disease, which were estimated to be over $736 million in 2000.[83] In 1998, ulcerative colitis patients had almost 500,000 physician office visits, 90,000 visits to either the emergency room or the outpatient clinic, and 47,000 inpatient stays, of which 53% were for primary diagnosis. As with Crohn's disease, hospital stays and drugs constitute the bulk of direct costs, which were estimated to be more than $404 million in 2000.[83] Other studies have confirmed the high costs of medical care for patients with Crohn's disease and ulcerative colitis.[137, 156, 157] The indirect costs (costs not directly related to medical care but encompassing other areas such as loss of wages and lost productivity) associated with inflammatory bowel disease are also high. Estimates for indirect costs in 2000 were almost $79 million for Crohn's disease and almost $38 million for ulcerative colitis.[83]

As with many chronic diseases, the intangible human costs of inflammatory bowel disease are very difficult to quantify. Patients with ulcerative colitis and Crohn's disease consistently demonstrate impairments in physical, social, and emotional function that are frequently underestimated by family and physicians and that may or may not be related to disease severity; these impairments include fears about life expectancy, family, employment, ability to carry out normal daily activities, surgery, cancer, side effects, flare-ups, treatment options, finances, and whether the patients' children were likely to get the disease.[158, 159]

There are several conclusions to be drawn from the information presented above:

- Inflammatory bowel diseases are costly and disabling disorders in which the primary pathology involves inflammation in the gastrointestinal tract.
- Inflammatory bowel diseases are associated with many diseases and dysfunctions involving essentially all body systems, including autoimmune diseases, highlighting the association between gut inflammation and systemic disease.

Gastrointestinal Inflammation and the Spondyloarthritides

Spondyloarthritis is a term used to describe any one of a group of autoimmune inflammatory joint diseases that have been separated, based on association with the HLA-B27 gene and clinical features, from rheumatoid arthritis. The classification and nomenclature have undergone changes over the years; these diseases were previously known as spondyloarthropathies, but the term spondyloarthritides is now preferred as it emphasizes the inflammatory nature of the disease process.[160] The spondyloarthritides are currently classified into the following categories: ankylosing spondylitis, reactive arthritis or Reiter's syndrome, arthritis/spondylitis that occurs in association with inflammatory bowel disease, arthritis/spondylitis that occurs in association with psoriasis, and undifferentiated spondyloarthritis, which has features specific for spondyloarthritis but does not fulfill the criteria for any of the defined diseases. In almost all cases, inflammatory back pain, with or without an accompanying asymmetrical arthritis, is the most prominent symptom.[161, 162]

Ankylosing spondylitis is the most frequent and severe of the spondyloarthritides, the prototype disease for these conditions.[163] The disease commonly starts in the second of third decade of life, and sacroiliitis is almost always the earliest recognized manifestation. Ankylosing spondylitis may evolve from a previously undifferentiated spondyloarthritis over the course of several years.[164] Irreversible damage to the sacroiliac joints occurs with time, leading in advanced cases to ossification and "bamboo spine" secondary to *osteoproliferation* that occurs after the initial bone destruction.[165] Hyperkyphosis is a particularly disturbing feature of advanced disease.[165, 166] The axial arthritis is usually associated with peripheral arthritis, enthesitis (inflammation of ligamentous attachments to bone), and anterior uveitis.[165] The peripheral arthritis is usually monarticular or oligoarticular and mainly affects the lower limbs.[165] Ankylosing spondylitis appears to be more common in men, in whom there is a different disease pattern, with the spine and pelvis being involved more commonly, whereas in women, peripheral disease is more common.[161]

The incidence and prevalence of ankylosing spondylitis correlate strongly with the presence of HLA-B27 in a population.[162, 165] Most epidemiological studies have been conducted in Europe among blood donors, and the prevalence in these studies ranges from 0% to 20% in HLA-B27-positive donors and from 0% to 3% in HLA-B27-negative donors. In a review[162] of several European studies, the prevalence of ankylosing spondylitis ranged from 0.14% to 1.8% (in the population with the highest prevalence of HLA-B27), and the prevalence of spondyloarthritis as a whole ranged from 0.3% to 1.73%. Studies reporting the prevalence of ankylosing spondylitis in the United States are scarce. One study compiled data from a variety of survey populations and calculated a prevalence of ankylosing spondylitis of 0.1% to 0.12% and a prevalence of spondyloarthritis in general as 0.21% in the U.S. population.[167]

While arthritis is certainly the main feature of spondyloarthritides, there are many other systemic dysfunctions associated with these diseases, as is clear from the categorization of some of them based on the association with other inflammatory diseases (see Table 1.3). Spondyloarthritides, then, like all the diseases discussed in this chapter, should be considered multisystem diseases; the classification system currently in place may be an inappropriate way to differentiate them.

Table 1.3—Comorbidities of Spondyloarthritides

- Inflammatory bowel disease in arthritis/spondylitis
- Psoriasis in arthritis/spondylitis
- Uveitis in arthritis/spondylitis
- Diabetes, hypertension, obesity, and hyperlipidemia in psoriatic arthritis[168]
- Pleuropulmonary involvement in ankylosing spondylitis[169, 170]
- Eye involvement in spondyloarthritides other than Reiter's syndrome[170]
- Subclinical gastrointestinal inflammation in ankylosing spondylitis[163]
- Low bone density, osteoporosis, and increased fracture rates in ankylosing spondylitis[165]
- Increased cardiovascular risk in all spondyloarthritides[171]

There is mounting evidence to suggest that gut inflammation plays a part in the pathogenesis of all the spondyloarthritides, not only those associated with inflammatory bowel disease.[130, 163, 165, 172] Subclinical gut inflammation (particularly ileitis) revealed by ileocolonoscopy has been found in up to 60% of ankylosing spondylitis patients,[172] as well as in patients with other forms of spondyloarthritis.[163] In ankylosing spondylitis patients, the prevalence of gut inflammation is higher in those with peripheral arthritis than in those without. Chronic inflammatory lesions on gut histology are associated with more advanced radiological sacroiliac disease and more destructive peripheral articular disease. And remission of joint inflammation has been found to be associated with remission of gut inflammation.[163]

In particular, evidence has been accumulating over the past 3 decades suggesting that *Klebsiella* infection of the gut (clinical or subclinical) may be a triggering or perpetuating factor in the pathophysiology of ankylosing spondylitis. In a recent review, Rashid and Ebringer[130] discussed the following evidence:

- Studies have showed a temporal relationship between acquisition of *Klebsiella* in the feces and the exacerbation of ankylosing spondylitis symptoms.
- Elevated serum levels of antibodies against *Klebsiella* have been found to be associated with a higher degree of gut inflammation in ankylosing spondylitis patients; the concentrations were higher in serum than in joints, suggesting that antibodies may be produced in nonarticular regions before gaining access to the joints.
- Molecular homology has been demonstrated between certain amino acid sequences in *Klebsiella* and HLA-B27 molecules.
- Antibodies to *Klebsiella* have been found in sera of HLA-B27-positive ankylosing spondylitis patients with acute anterior uveitis.

The authors of this review[130] suggested that repeated (probably subclinical) infections with *Klebsiella* are the probable triggering events in the pathogenesis of ankylosing spondylitis. Providing even further evidence of the centrality of events in the gastrointestinal tract to the pathogenesis of spondyloarthritis, several studies have led researchers to suggest a possible link between Crohn's disease and ankylosing spondylitis,[160] perhaps via *Klebsiella*.[131]

There is little reported information on the healthcare costs associated with ankylosing spondylitis, and studies from different countries are difficult to compare.[166] There is more information on the decreases in physical functioning and quality of life in ankylosing spondylitis patients. The decrease in physical functioning is similar to, or worse than, that seen in rheumatoid arthritis patients.[166] Patients have to deal with pain, functional disability, dependency, and income loss, all of which can negatively affect quality of life.[166] In a longitudinal study of ankylosing spondylitis patients, the most prevalent quality of life concerns included stiffness, pain, fatigue, poor sleep, appearance, worry about the future, and medication side effects.[173] In virtually all studies that assess quality of life in spondyloarthritis patients, quality of life is strongly related to functionality; as function decreases, so does quality of life.[174, 175] In addition, the presence of comorbid conditions contributes to decreased quality of life in these patients.[166]

The information presented above reminds us that:

- The spondyloarthritides are disabling, chronic autoimmune diseases, with accompanying systemic manifestations, which occur at a relatively young age. In addition to the joints, multiple other organ systems are involved.
- Current classification systems of the spondyloarthritides may be inappropriate, as the pathogenesis may be similar across groups.
- There is significant evidence to suggest a role for gastrointestinal inflammation, in particular related to *Klebsiella* infection, in the pathogenesis of ankylosing spondylitis.

Gastrointestinal Inflammation and Cancer

While there are clearly many factors involved in the etiology of cancer, the role of chronic inflammation is being increasingly recognized.[124, 155, 176, 177] About 560,000 Americans were expected to die of cancer in 2007—more than 1,500 people per day.[178] Since 1999, cancer has surpassed heart disease as the number one killer of people under the age of 85.[179] It was estimated that 1.5 million new cases of cancer would be diagnosed in 2007 in the United States,[178] including these cancers of the gastrointestinal tract:

- The incidence of esophageal adenocarcinoma in the United States tripled between 1976 and 1990.[180] Esophageal cancer accounts for 1% of all cancers diagnosed in the United States.[87] Adenocarcinoma now accounts for more than 50% of esophageal cancers and afflicts about 10,000 people every year; prognosis is poor, with an overall 5-year survival rate of only about 10%.[180] The rate has also been rising in Western Europe.[181]
- Gastric cancer is the fourth most common cancer in the world; almost two-thirds of these cases occur in the developing world, with particularly high rates in Japan (especially in males), throughout East Asia, and in Central and South America.[92, 182] It was estimated that there would be 21,260 new cases of gastric cancer, of which 90% are adenocarcinomas,[88] in the United States in 2007 (13,000 in men and 8,260 in women) and that 11,210 people would die of this disease (6,610 men and 4,600 women).[178]
- Colorectal cancer was expected to be the third most common new cancer diagnosis in 2007, as well as the third leading cause of cancer death. It was estimated that colon cancer would cause an estimated 52,180 deaths in the United States in 2007 and that there would be 112,340 new cases.[178]

Chronic activation of the immune system by infective agents is a well-described precursor of cancer; examples include the association between *H. pylori* and stomach cancer, schistosomiasis and bladder cancer, and hepatitis viruses and liver cancer.[176] Esophageal cancer appears to have a pathogenetic link to inflammation of the gastrointestinal tract. While several factors are implicated in the etiology of esophageal adenocarcinoma, gastroesophageal reflux disease appears to be the most important risk factor.[180] Chronic gastroesophageal reflux leads to chronic irritation and inflammation of the esophageal mucosa, resulting in inflammation-stimulated hyperplasia, metaplasia, multifocal dysplasia, carcinoma *in situ*, and eventually invasive adenocarcinoma.[180] The presence of Barrett's esophagus (a condition characterized by abnormal "tongues" of salmon-colored mucosa extending proximally from the gastroesophageal junction into the normally pale esophageal mucosa[183]) has been viewed as a crucial link between reflux and carcinogenesis. However, in one study, Barrett's esophagus was present in only 62% of esophageal adenocarcinoma patients while the risk of esophageal adenocarcinoma was found to be 8 times higher among persons in whom heartburn and/or regurgitation occurred at least once a week than in those without these symptoms. Thus, the authors hypothesized that it is esophageal reflux itself, with its associated chronic inflammation (with or without Barrett's esophagus), that may be the crucial factor in cancer pathogenesis.[181]

Gastric adenocarcinoma is another cancer that appears to have a direct pathogenetic link to gut inflammation. Although several factors obviously influence an individual's predisposition to develop gastric cancer,[88] or any cancer, recent evidence suggests that inflammation is an important predisposing factor,[101] particularly because of the association with *H. pylori*.[101] Briefly, *H. pylori* is believed to induce proinflammatory responses in gastric epithelial cells attempting to clear the host of infection. Chronic inflammation results in increased cytokine production that mobilizes and recruits bone marrow-derived stem cells from the circulation. Epithelial metaplasia and dysplasia, and eventually cancer, follow.[101] In addition, it has been postulated that the loss of gastric acid secretion accompanying *H. pylori*-associated gastritis allows overgrowth of other bacterial species that may also be implicated in the progression to adenocarcinoma.[101]

Colon cancer is also associated pathogenetically with chronic gut inflammation. In fact, inflammatory bowel disease is considered a major risk factor in the development of colorectal cancer.[155] Interestingly, there are studies suggesting that colon cancers unrelated to inflammatory bowel disease may have an inflammatory pathogenetic component.[184]

A few recent articles examined the possible association between gut inflammation and cancers occurring outside the gastrointestinal tract. In one study, the authors suggested that chronic gut inflammation may be implicated in the causation of breast cancer.[177] These researchers serendipitously discovered that mice infected with *Helicobacter hepaticus* developed mammary carcinoma within 4 to 6 weeks of infection.[177] It also has been suggested that chronic inflammation secondary to antigenic stimulation (such as that seen with *H. pylori* colonization of the stomach) is involved in the pathogenesis of MALT lymphomas[124] (see the Clinical Pearl above); chronic antigenic stimulation is thought to trigger inflammatory responses by attracting neutrophils, which release genotoxic reactive oxygen species.[124] Inflammatory bowel disease has been posed as a risk factor for lymphoma.[185]

NIH estimated that in 2006, cancer cost more than $263 billion in the United States, including over $78 billion in direct medical costs, almost $18 billion in indirect costs, and more than $110 billion in indirect mortality costs (costs of lost productivity due to premature death).[186] Newer anticancer drugs contribute in large measure to the direct costs of cancer care. A 2007 article reported that the cost for a 6-month course of cancer treatment with fluorouracil plus leucovorin (FU/LV), the only available treatment for colorectal cancer prior to 1996, was $96; treatment with combinations that include newer cytotoxic agents such as irinotecan brings the cost up to somewhere between $20,000 and $30,000. A 6-month course of cetuximab (administered weekly for colorectal cancer, as well as head and neck cancer) costs a staggering $52,131.[187] Interestingly, the increased survival with many of these newer agents can be measured in months only; the aggregate drug cost for treatment of patients with metastatic colorectal cancer is $150,000 to $200,000 for an additional year of survival when compared with treatment with FU/LV alone.[187] The high cost of cancer treatment has a profound impact on patients.[188]

There are several conclusions to be drawn from the information presented above:

- Cancer, a costly and burdensome disease, is a major cause of mortality in the United States, Europe, and around the world.
- There is evidence that chronic inflammation of the gut is implicated in the pathogenesis of several cancers of the gastrointestinal tract and possibly of other cancers of non-epithelial cells that occur outside the gastrointestinal tract.
- Reduction of inflammation in the gastrointestinal tract should be a primary goal in cancer prevention.

Emerging Issues in Gastrointestinal Inflammation: Irritable Bowel Syndrome

While there is abundant evidence linking gastrointestinal inflammation with the diseases and dysfunctions discussed above, there is an emerging, although as yet poorly defined, relationship between gut inflammation and other disorders, including irritable bowel syndrome. Here we will briefly discuss the emerging evidence for (and against) the role of gut inflammation in the pathogenesis of this disorder.

Historically, the term *functional gastrointestinal disorder* was used to separate ulcerative colitis and Crohn's disease from various combinations of chronic or recurrent gastrointestinal symptoms that could not be explained by established structural or biochemical abnormalities.[189,190,191] This term covers a very broad spectrum of disorders,[191] and the most frequently investigated are irritable bowel syndrome, dyspepsia, constipation, and functional esophageal disorders.[189] We will concentrate here on irritable bowel syndrome, the most common diagnosis made by gastroenterologists in the United States.[192]

Irritable bowel syndrome is a clinical diagnosis based on the presence of abdominal discomfort associated with a change in stool frequency that originated at least 6 months prior to diagnosis and that has been active (i.e., met the diagnostic criteria) for at least 3 months.[193] Although the diagnosis is often difficult, most authors agree that it should be based on the combination of symptoms that meet the Rome criteria, a physical gastrointestinal exam, and screening procedures (including blood tests, endoscopic procedures, barium enemas, and ultrasound) performed by the clinician to rule out "structural" diseases.[194,195]

Table 1.4—Rome III Diagnostic Criteria for Irritable Bowel Syndrome

At least 3 months, with onset at least 6 months previously, of recurrent abdominal pain or discomfort* associated with two or more of the following:

- Improvement with defecation
- Onset associated with a change in frequency of stool
- Onset associated with a change in form (appearance) of stool

*Discomfort means an uncomfortable sensation not described as pain.

It has been estimated that between 10% and 15% of people in North America have irritable bowel syndrome,[196] while the prevalence of irritable bowel syndrome around the world ranges from 0.8% to 28%.[189] Irritable bowel syndrome is more common in females[189] (or at least women appear more likely to seek medical care for their irritable bowel syndrome[197]), less common in the elderly,[189] and more common in upper-socioeconomic groups.[198] In 1998, there were 3.65 million physician office visits for irritable bowel syndrome,[83] and it is estimated that the syndrome accounts for 12% of primary care visits.[195] Irritable bowel syndrome patients make twice as many healthcare visits per year as age-matched controls.[199]

Direct costs related to irritable bowel syndrome, including inpatient and outpatient utilization and prescription medication use, were estimated to be greater than $1.7 billion in 2000,[83] and some estimates of annual direct costs in the United States are as high as $10 billion.[200] Irritable bowel syndrome patients have a high rate of unnecessary surgeries, such as cholecystectomy, hysterectomy, appendectomy, and back surgery, related in large part to symptom overlap with other disorders and incorrect diagnosis,[198] and these surgeries almost certainly contribute to the high direct costs involved in treatment of irritable bowel syndrome.

Indirect costs have been estimated to account for most of the financial burden associated with irritable bowel syndrome, in part because the syndrome largely affects people during their most productive years.[201] Estimated indirect costs of irritable bowel syndrome based on days missed and average wages lost were estimated to exceed $20 billion in 2000.[83] When we also consider the fact that only about 25% of people with irritable bowel syndrome seek medical help,[202] we can begin to appreciate the enormous burden placed on individuals, healthcare systems, and societies by this syndrome. Indeed, a review[200] noted that total costs associated with irritable bowel syndrome are greater than costs associated with asthma and migraine and comparable to costs associated with hypertension and congestive heart failure. The negative impact of irritable bowel syndrome on quality of life is also very significant,[203] similar to that in patients with other long-term episodic disorders such as migraine, asthma, and gastroesophageal reflux disease.[204]

Approximately 50% of irritable bowel syndrome patients have at least one comorbid symptom,[199] challenging the assumption that irritable bowel syndrome is a distinct lower gastrointestinal disease. Patients with irritable bowel syndrome frequently report symptoms from other parts of the gastrointestinal tract,[198, 199, 205] leading at least one researcher to question the wisdom of continuing to use complex classification systems such as the Rome criteria based purely on symptoms.[205] Extraintestinal comorbidities are also very common in irritable bowel syndrome patients; a review[199] of studies dealing with comorbidity found that 78% of primary care visits made by irritable bowel syndrome patients were for non-gastrointestinal symptoms and that 66% of excess costs incurred by irritable bowel syndrome patients were for non-gastrointestinal problems. Comorbidities include depression and anxiety, fatigue, cold intolerance, sleep disturbances, musculoskeletal pain, headache, and other symptoms consistent with a diagnosis of fibromyalgia or chronic fatigue syndrome; many patients also report symptoms consistent with temporomandibular joint disorder, and chronic pelvic pain has been reported in a significant number of women with irritable bowel syndrome.[199, 206] Other symptoms reported by irritable bowel syndrome patients include shortness of breath and wheezing.[198, 199, 206]

Table 1.5—Irritable Bowel Syndrome Comorbidities[199]

Psychiatric disorders (major depression, anxiety, somatoform disorders)—occur in up to 94% of irritable bowel syndrome patients
Fibromyalgia—49% have irritable bowel syndrome
Chronic fatigue syndrome—51% have irritable bowel syndrome
Temporomandibular joint disorder—64% have irritable bowel syndrome
Chronic pelvic pain—50% have irritable bowel syndrome

Several factors have been implicated in the etiology of irritable bowel syndrome, including genetic predisposition,[198] altered bowel motility, visceral hypersensitivity, alterations in bacterial composition (especially in the small bowel), psychosocial disturbances, neurotransmitter imbalance, infection, increased gut permeability, and inflammation.[195, 199, 207-210] Of particular interest for our purposes is evidence that inflammation is present in the enteric mucosa of irritable bowel syndrome patients.[195, 208, 209, 211] It has been well documented that there is a subset of irritable bowel syndrome patients who have had previous acute gastroenteritis,[189, 198, 208] and there is evidence that gastrointestinal inflammatory changes are present in these patients[208]; inefficient downregulation of inflammatory responses to infection is thought to be implicated.[208, 209] Recent research, however, suggests that inflammatory changes are present in the colonic mucosa of patients with other forms of irritable bowel syndrome, not only in post-infectious cases. Several studies (summarized in a recent review[208]) found mast cells and lymphocytes in the gastrointestinal mucosa in a wide variety of subtypes of irritable bowel syndrome, as well as in patients with post-infectious disease. Furthermore, increased gut permeability has been found in patients with diarrhea-predominant irritable bowel syndrome, with the defect being more severe than in patients with post-infectious disease.[212]

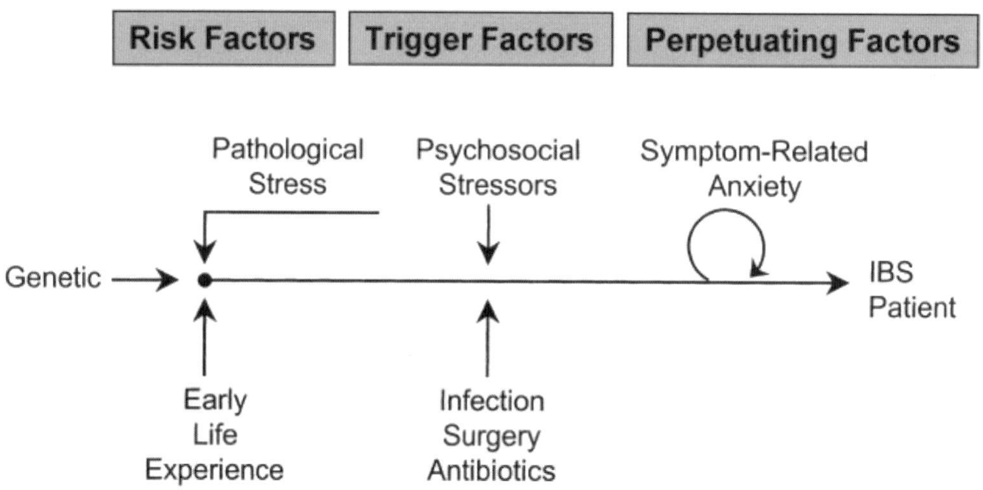

Figure 1.2—Development and Modulation of Irritable Bowel Syndrome Symptoms

Source: Mayer EA, Naliboff BD, Chang L, Coutinho SV. V. stress and irritable bowel syndrome. *Am J Physiol Gastrointest Liver Physiol.* 2001;280:G519-524. ©2001, The American Physiological Society. Used with permission.

The full significance of these findings is as yet unclear, and the relevance to the etiology of extraintestinal manifestations of irritable bowel syndrome is currently unknown. Indeed, there is no unifying hypothesis that explains both irritable bowel syndrome and its comorbidities.[195, 199] At least one researcher has postulated that inflammation may be the final common pathway in all the functional gastrointestinal disorders.[205] Future research will no doubt continue to shed light on that hypothesis and the pathogenesis of this ubiquitous disorder.

Clinical Pearl:

Irritable bowel syndrome patients who experience increased symptoms from the conventional high-fiber diet may be suffering from a gut fermentation syndrome provoked by small bowel bacterial overgrowth. These patients may benefit from reducing fiber and carbohydrates and adding antimicrobial drugs or herbs.

Summary

From the information presented in this chapter, it is clear that gastrointestinal inflammation is associated with (and sometimes directly responsible for) a wide variety of debilitating disorders and dysfunctions, both within the gastrointestinal tract itself and in virtually all organ systems in the body. The ways in which gastrointestinal immune dysregulation and its effects throughout the body can present, however, can be a challenge to clinicians. Frequently, presenting signs, symptoms, and disease processes may yield few clues that the primary pathology lies in the gut. It is crucial that clinicians are aware of the wide-ranging effects of gut inflammation and the myriad ways in which it can present. Addressing gut immune dysregulation and inflammation is a key factor in improving assessment, treatment, and prevention of a wide range of systemic disease processes.

References

1. Takahashi I, Kiyono H. Gut as the largest immunologic tissue. *JPEN J Parenter Enteral Nutr.* 1999;23:S7-12.
2. Macdonald TT, Monteleone G. Immunity, inflammation, and allergy in the gut. *Science.* 2005;307:1920-1925.
3. Farrell RJ, Kelly CP. Celiac sprue. *N Engl J Med.* 2002;346:180-188.
4. Lee SK, Green PH. Celiac sprue (the great modern-day imposter). *Curr Opin Rheumatol.* 2006;18:101-107.
5. Hadjivassiliou M, Williamson CA, Woodroofe N. The immunology of gluten sensitivity: beyond the gut. *Trends Immunol.* 2004;25:578-582.
6. Marsh MN. Gluten, major histocompatibility complex, and the small intestine. A molecular and immunobiologic approach to the spectrum of gluten sensitivity ('celiac sprue'). *Gastroenterology.* 1992;102:330-354.
7. Fasano A. Systemic autoimmune disorders in celiac disease. *Curr Opin Gastroenterol.* 2006;22:674-679.
8. van Heel DA, West J. Recent advances in coeliac disease. *Gut.* 2006;55:1037-1046.
9. McManus R, Kelleher D. Celiac disease--the villain unmasked? *N Engl J Med.* 2003;348:2573-2574.
10. Nieuwenhuizen WF, Pieters RH, Knippels LM, Jansen MC, Koppelman SJ. Is Candida albicans a trigger in the onset of coeliac disease? *Lancet.* 2003;361:2152-2154.
11. Fasano A. European and North American populations should be screened for coeliac disease. *Gut.* 2003;52:168-169.
12. Fasano A. Celiac disease--how to handle a clinical chameleon. *N Engl J Med.* 2003;348:2568-2570.
13. Kaukinen K, Peraaho M, Collin P, et al. Small-bowel mucosal transglutaminase 2-specific IgA deposits in coeliac disease without villous atrophy: a prospective and randomized clinical study. *Scand J Gastroenterol.* 2005;40:564-572.
14. Tursi A, Brandimarte G. The symptomatic and histologic response to a gluten-free diet in patients with borderline enteropathy. *J Clin Gastroenterol.* 2003;36:13-17.
15. Antonioli DA. Celiac disease: a progress report. *Mod Pathol.* 2003;16:342-346.
16. Abrams JA, Diamond B, Rotterdam H, Green PH. Seronegative celiac disease: increased prevalence with lesser degrees of villous atrophy. *Dig Dis Sci.* 2004;49:546-550.
17. NIH Consensus Development Conference on Celiac Disease. *NIH Consens State Sci Statements.* 2004;21:1-23.
18. Rewers M. Epidemiology of celiac disease: what are the prevalence, incidence, and progression of celiac disease? *Gastroenterology.* 2005;128: S47-51.
19. Bingley PJ, Williams AJ, Norcross AJ, et al. Undiagnosed coeliac disease at age seven: population based prospective birth cohort study. *Bmj.* 2004;328:322-323.
20. Maki M, Mustalahti K, Kokkonen J, et al. Prevalence of Celiac disease among children in Finland. *N Engl J Med.* 2003;348:2517-2524.
21. West J, Logan RF, Hill PG, et al. Seroprevalence, correlates, and characteristics of undetected coeliac disease in England. *Gut.* 2003;52:960-965.
22. Fasano A, Berti I, Gerarduzzi T, et al. Prevalence of celiac disease in at-risk and not-at-risk groups in the United States: a large multicenter study. *Arch Intern Med.* 2003;163:286-292.
23. Cranney A, Zarkadas M, Graham ID, et al. The Canadian Celiac Health Survey. *Dig Dis Sci.* 2007;52:1087-1095.
24. Green PHR, Stavropoulos SN, Panagi SG, et al. Characteristics of adult celiac disease in the USA: results of a national survey. *Am J Gastroenterol.* 2001;96:126-131.
25. Barton SH, Kelly DG, Murray JA. Nutritional deficiencies in celiac disease. *Gastroenterol Clin North Am.* 2007;36:93-108.

26. Maiuri L, Ciacci C, Ricciardelli I, et al. Association between innate response to gliadin and activation of pathogenic T cells in coeliac disease. *Lancet.* 2003;362:30-37.
27. Forsberg G, Fahlgren A, Horstedt P, Hammarstrom S, Hernell O, Hammarstrom ML. Presence of bacteria and innate immunity of intestinal epithelium in childhood celiac disease. *Am J Gastroenterol.* 2004;99:894-904.
28. Stene LC, Honeyman MC, Hoffenberg EJ, et al. Rotavirus infection frequency and risk of celiac disease autoimmunity in early childhood: a longitudinal study. *Am J Gastroenterol.* 2006;101:2333-2340.
29. Collin P, Reunala T. Recognition and management of the cutaneous manifestations of celiac disease: a guide for dermatologists. *Am J Clin Dermatol.* 2003;4:13-20.
30. Hadjivassiliou M, Boscolo S, Davies-Jones GA, et al. The humoral response in the pathogenesis of gluten ataxia. *Neurology.* 2002;58:1221-1226.
31. Halfdanarson TR, Litzow MR, Murray JA. Hematologic manifestations of celiac disease. *Blood.* 2007;109:412-421.
32. Lubrano E, Ciacci C, Ames PR, Mazzacca G, Oriente P, Scarpa R. The arthritis of coeliac disease: prevalence and pattern in 200 adult patients. *Br J Rheumatol.* 1996;35:1314-1318.
33. Corazza GR, Di Stefano M, Maurino E, Bai JC. Bones in coeliac disease: diagnosis and treatment. *Best Pract Res Clin Gastroenterol.* 2005;19:453-465.
34. Bushara KO. Neurologic presentation of celiac disease. *Gastroenterology.* 2005;128:S92-97.
35. Sategna-Guidetti C, Volta U, Ciacci C, et al. Prevalence of thyroid disorders in untreated adult celiac disease patients and effect of gluten withdrawal: an Italian multicenter study. *Am J Gastroenterol.* 2001;96:751-757.
36. Carta MG, Hardoy MC, Boi MF, Mariotti S, Carpiniello B, Usai P. Association between panic disorder, major depressive disorder and celiac disease: a possible role of thyroid autoimmunity. *J Psychosom Res.* 2002;53:789-793.
37. Abdo A, Meddings J, Swain M. Liver abnormalities in celiac disease. *Clin Gastroenterol Hepatol.* 2004;2:107-112.
38. Wierink CD, van Diermen DE, Aartman IH, Heymans HS. Dental enamel defects in children with coeliac disease. *Int J Paediatr Dent.* 2007;17:163-168.
39. Abenavoli L, Leggio L, Gasbarrini G, Addolorato G. Celiac disease and skin: Psoriasis association. *World J Gastroenterol.* 2007;13:2138-2139.
40. Cronin CC, Shanahan F. Insulin-dependent diabetes mellitus and coeliac disease. *Lancet.* 1997;349:1096-1097.
41. Ludvigsson JF, Ludvigsson J, Ekbom A, Montgomery SM. Celiac disease and risk of subsequent type 1 diabetes: a general population cohort study of children and adolescents. *Diabetes Care.* 2006;29:2483-2488.
42. Brousse N, Meijer JW. Malignant complications of coeliac disease. *Best Pract Res Clin Gastroenterol.* 2005;19:401-412.
43. Ventura A, Martelossi S. Dental enamel defects and coeliac disease. *Arch Dis Child.* 1997;77:91.
44. Jones DS, ed. *Textbook of Functional Medicine.* Gig Harbor, WA: The Institute for Functional Medicine; 2005.
45. Smellie WS, Wilson D, McNulty CA, et al. Best practice in primary care pathology: review 1. *J Clin Pathol.* 2005;58:1016-1024.
46. Mahmud FH, Murray JA, Kudva YC, et al. Celiac disease in type 1 diabetes mellitus in a North American community: prevalence, serologic screening, and clinical features. *Mayo Clin Proc.* 2005;80:1429-1434.
47. Barera G, Bonfanti R, Viscardi M, et al. Occurrence of celiac disease after onset of type 1 diabetes: a 6-year prospective longitudinal study. *Pediatrics.* 2002;109:833-838.
48. Hansen D, Brock-Jacobsen B, Lund E, et al. Clinical benefit of a gluten-free diet in type 1 diabetic children with screening-detected celiac disease: a population-based screening study with 2 years' follow-up. *Diabetes Care.* 2006;29:2452-2456.
49. Ziegler AG, Schmid S, Huber D, Hummel M, Bonifacio E. Early infant feeding and risk of developing type 1 diabetes-associated autoantibodies. *Jama.* 2003;290:1721-1728.
50. Ventura A, Neri E, Ughi C, Leopaldi A, Citta A, Not T. Gluten-dependent diabetes-related and thyroid-related autoantibodies in patients with celiac disease. *J Pediatr.* 2000;137:263-265.
51. Berti I, Trevisiol C, Tommasini A, et al. Usefulness of screening program for celiac disease in autoimmune thyroiditis. *Dig Dis Sci.* 2000;45:403-406.
52. Counsell CE, Taha A, Ruddell WS. Coeliac disease and autoimmune thyroid disease. *Gut.* 1994;35:844-846.
53. Ch'ng CL, Biswas M, Benton A, Jones MK, Kingham JG. Prospective screening for coeliac disease in patients with Graves' hyperthyroidism using anti-gliadin and tissue transglutaminase antibodies. *Clin Endocrinol (Oxf).* 2005;62:303-306.
54. da Silva Kotze LM, Nisihara RM, da Rosa Utiyama SR, Piovezan GC, Kotze LR. Thyroid disorders in Brazilian patients with celiac disease. *J Clin Gastroenterol.* 2006;40:33-36.
55. Ihara M, Makino F, Sawada H, et al. Gluten sensitivity in Japanese patients with adult-onset cerebellar ataxia. *Intern Med.* 2006;45:135-140.
56. Goldacre MJ, Wotton CJ, Seagroatt V, Yeates D. Cancers and immune related diseases associated with Down's syndrome: a record linkage study. *Arch Dis Child.* 2004;89:1014-1017.
57. Alaedini A, Okamoto H, Briani C, et al. Immune cross-reactivity in celiac disease: anti-gliadin antibodies bind to neuronal synapsin I. *J Immunol.* 2007;178:6590-6595.
58. Fox PC. Autoimmune diseases and Sjogren's syndrome: an autoimmune exocrinopathy. *Ann N Y Acad Sci.* 2007;1098:15-21.
59. Szodoray P, Barta Z, Lakos G, Szakall S, Zeher M. Coeliac disease in Sjogren's syndrome--a study of 111 Hungarian patients. *Rheumatol Int.* 2004;24:278-282.
60. Iltanen S, Collin P, Korpela M, et al. Celiac disease and markers of celiac disease latency in patients with primary Sjogren's syndrome. *Am J Gastroenterol.* 1999;94:1042-1046.
61. Luft LM, Barr SG, Martin LO, Chan EK, Fritzler MJ. Autoantibodies to tissue transglutaminase in Sjogren's syndrome and related rheumatic diseases. *J Rheumatol.* 2003;30:2613-2619.
62. Kassan SS, Moutsopoulos HM. Clinical manifestations and early diagnosis of Sjogren syndrome. *Arch Intern Med.* 2004;164:1275-1284.
63. Roblin X, Helluwaert F, Bonaz B. Celiac disease must be evaluated in patients with Sjogren syndrome. *Arch Intern Med.* 2004;164:2387.
64. Karpati S. Dermatitis herpetiformis: close to unravelling a disease. *J Dermatol Sci.* 2004;34:83-90.
65. Wasserman D, Guzman-Sanchez DA, Scott K, McMichael A. Alopecia areata. *Int J Dermatol.* 2007;46:121-131.
66. Addolorato G, Parente A, de Lorenzi G, et al. Rapid regression of psoriasis in a coeliac patient after gluten-free diet. A case report and review of the literature. *Digestion.* 2003;68:9-12.
67. Liu Y, Krueger JG, Bowcock AM. Psoriasis: genetic associations and immune system changes. *Genes Immun.* 2007;8:1-12.
68. Michaelsson G, Gerden B, Hagforsen E, et al. Psoriasis patients with antibodies to gliadin can be improved by a gluten-free diet. *Br J Dermatol.* 2000;142:44-51.

69. Ojetti V, Aguilar Sanchez J, Guerriero C, et al. High prevalence of celiac disease in psoriasis. *Am J Gastroenterol.* 2003;98:2574-2575.
70. Fessatou S, Kostaki M, Karpathios T. Coeliac disease and alopecia areata in childhood. *J Paediatr Child Health.* 2003;39:152-154.
71. Barbato M, Viola F, Grillo R, et al. Alopecia and coeliac disease: report of two patients showing response to gluten-free diet. *Clin Exp Dermatol.* 1998;23:236-237.
72. Naveh Y, Rosenthal E, Ben-Arieh Y, Etzioni A. Celiac disease-associated alopecia in childhood. *J Pediatr.* 1999;134:362-364.
73. Hadjivassiliou M, Grunewald RA, Lawden M, Davies-Jones GA, Powell T, Smith CM. Headache and CNS white matter abnormalities associated with gluten sensitivity. *Neurology.* 2001;56:385-388.
74. Waeber C, Moskowitz MA. Migraine as an inflammatory disorder. *Neurology.* 2005;64:S9-15.
75. Raison CL, Capuron L, Miller AH. Cytokines sing the blues: inflammation and the pathogenesis of depression. *Trends Immunol.* 2006;27:24-31.
76. Stagi S, Giani T, Simonini G, Falcini F. Thyroid function, autoimmune thyroiditis and coeliac disease in juvenile idiopathic arthritis. *Rheumatology (Oxford).* 2005;44:517-520.
77. Holmes GK, Prior P, Lane MR, Pope D, Allan RN. Malignancy in coeliac disease--effect of a gluten free diet. *Gut.* 1989;30:333-338.
78. Anderson LA, McMillan SA, Watson RG, et al. Malignancy and mortality in a population-based cohort of patients with coeliac disease or "gluten sensitivity". *World J Gastroenterol.* 2007;13:146-151.
79. Johnston SD, Watson RG. Small bowel lymphoma in unrecognized coeliac disease: a cause for concern? *Eur J Gastroenterol Hepatol.* 2000;12:645-648.
80. Catassi C, Bearzi I, Holmes GK. Association of celiac disease and intestinal lymphomas and other cancers. *Gastroenterology.* 2005;128:S79-86.
81. Kumar PJ. European and North American populations should be screened for coeliac disease. *Gut.* 2003;52:170-171.
82. Zipser RD, Patel S, Yahya KZ, Baisch DW, Monarch E. Presentations of adult celiac disease in a nationwide patient support group. *Dig Dis Sci.* 2003;48:761-764.
83. The American Gastroenterological Association. The Burden of Gastrointestinal Diseases. http://www.gastro.org/wmspage.cfm?parm1=3234. Accessed Feb. 12, 2008.
84. Freston JW. Management of peptic ulcers: emerging issues. *World J Surg.* 2000;24:250-255.
85. Pasceri V, Patti G, Cammarota G, Pristipino C, Richichi G, Di Sciascio G. Virulent strains of Helicobacter pylori and vascular diseases: a meta-analysis. *Am Heart J.* 2006;151:1215-1222.
86. Chan FK, Leung WK. Peptic-ulcer disease. *Lancet.* 2002;360:933-941.
87. Gallo A, Cha C. Updates on esophageal and gastric cancers. *World J Gastroenterol.* 2006;12:3237-3242.
88. Kelley JR, Duggan JM. Gastric cancer epidemiology and risk factors. *J Clin Epidemiol.* 2003;56:1-9.
89. Uemura N, Okamoto S, Yamamoto S, et al. Helicobacter pylori infection and the development of gastric cancer. *N Engl J Med.* 2001;345:784-789.
90. Ferrucci PF, Zucca E. Primary gastric lymphoma pathogenesis and treatment: what has changed over the past 10 years? *Br J Haematol.* 2007;136:521-538.
91. Malaty HM. Epidemiology of Helicobacter pylori infection. *Best Pract Res Clin Gastroenterol.* 2007;21:205-214.
92. Parkin DM. International variation. *Oncogene.* 2004;23:6329-6340.
93. Kountouras J, Zavos C, Chatzopoulos D. Primary open-angle glaucoma: pathophysiology and treatment. *Lancet.* 2004;364:1311-1312.
94. Barabino A. Helicobacter pylori-related iron deficiency anemia: a review. *Helicobacter.* 2002;7:71-75.
95. Franceschi F, Sepulveda AR, Gasbarrini A, et al. Cross-reactivity of anti-CagA antibodies with vascular wall antigens: possible pathogenic link between Helicobacter pylori infection and atherosclerosis. *Circulation.* 2002;106:430-434.
96. Kodama M, Kitadai Y, Ito M, et al. Immune response to CagA protein is associated with improved platelet count after Helicobacter pylori eradication in patients with idiopathic thrombocytopenic purpura. *Helicobacter.* 2007;12:36-42.
97. Weller C, Oxlade N, Dobbs SM, Dobbs RJ, Charlett A, Bjarnason IT. Role of inflammation in gastrointestinal tract in aetiology and pathogenesis of idiopathic parkinsonism. *FEMS Immunol Med Microbiol.* 2005;44:129-135.
98. Gasbarrini A, Franceschi F, Armuzzi A, et al. Extradigestive manifestations of Helicobacter pylori gastric infection. *Gut.* 1999;45 Suppl 1:I9-I12.
99. Carloni E, Cremonini F, Di Caro S, et al. Helicobacter pylori-related extradigestive diseases and effects of eradication therapy. *Dig Liver Dis.* 2000;32 Suppl 3:S214-216.
100. Velin D, Michetti P. Immunology of Helicobacter pylori infection. *Digestion.* 2006;73:116-123.
101. Fox JG, Wang TC. Inflammation, atrophy, and gastric cancer. *J Clin Invest.* 2007;117:60-69.
102. Franceschi F, Gasbarrini A. Helicobacter pylori and extragastric diseases. *Best Pract Res Clin Gastroenterol.* 2007;21:325-334.
103. Ameriso SF, Fridman EA, Leiguarda RC, Sevlever GE. Detection of Helicobacter pylori in human carotid atherosclerotic plaques. *Stroke.* 2001;32:385-391.
104. Huber MR, Kumar S, Tefferi A. Treatment advances in adult immune thrombocytopenic purpura. *Ann Hematol.* 2003;82:723-737.
105. Campuzano-Maya G. Proof of an Association between Helicobacter pylori and Idiopathic Thrombocytopenic Purpura in Latin America. *Helicobacter.* 2007;12:265-273.
106. Stasi R, Rossi Z, Stipa E, Amadori S, Newland AC, Provan D. Helicobacter pylori eradication in the management of patients with idiopathic thrombocytopenic purpura. *Am J Med.* 2005;118:414-419.
107. Sato R, Murakami K, Watanabe K, et al. Effect of Helicobacter pylori eradication on platelet recovery in patients with chronic idiopathic thrombocytopenic purpura. *Arch Intern Med.* 2004;164:1904-1907.
108. Inaba T, Mizuno M, Take S, et al. Eradication of Helicobacter pylori increases platelet count in patients with idiopathic thrombocytopenic purpura in Japan. *Eur J Clin Invest.* 2005;35:214-219.
109. Suzuki T, Matsushima M, Masui A, et al. Effect of Helicobacter pylori eradication in patients with chronic idiopathic thrombocytopenic purpura-a randomized controlled trial. *Am J Gastroenterol.* 2005;100:1265-1270.
110. Kostaki M, Fessatou S, Karpathios T. Refractory iron-deficiency anaemia due to silent Helicobacter pylori gastritis in children. *Eur J Pediatr.* 2003;162:177-179.
111. Ashorn M, Ruuska T, Makipernaa A. Helicobacter pylori and iron deficiency anaemia in children. *Scand J Gastroenterol.* 2001;36:701-705.
112. Russo-Mancuso G, Branciforte F, Licciardello M, La Spina M. Iron deficiency anemia as the only sign of infection with Helicobacter pylori: a report of 9 pediatric cases. *Int J Hematol.* 2003;78:429-431.
113. Choe YH, Kim SK, Hong YC. The relationship between Helicobacter pylori infection and iron deficiency: seroprevalence study in 937 pubescent children. *Arch Dis Child.* 2003;88:178.
114. Ferrara M, Coppola L, Coppola A, Capozzi L. Iron deficiency in childhood and adolescence: retrospective review. *Hematology.* 2006;11:183-186.

115. Choe YH, Kim SK, Son BK, Lee DH, Hong YC, Pai SH. Randomized placebo-controlled trial of Helicobacter pylori eradication for iron-deficiency anemia in preadolescent children and adolescents. *Helicobacter.* 1999;4:135-139.
116. Annibale B, Capurso G, Lahner E, et al. Concomitant alterations in intragastric pH and ascorbic acid concentration in patients with Helicobacter pylori gastritis and associated iron deficiency anaemia. *Gut.* 2003;52:496-501.
117. Otasevic L, Walduck A, Meyer TF, et al. Helicobacter pylori infection in anterior uveitis. *Infection.* 2005;33:82-85.
118. Otasevic L, Zlatanovic G, Stanojevic-Paovic A, et al. Helicobacter pylori: an underestimated factor in acute anterior uveitis and spondyloarthropathies? *Ophthalmologica.* 2007;221:6-13.
119. Weller C, Charlett A, Oxlade NL, et al. Role of chronic infection and inflammation in the gastrointestinal tract in the etiology and pathogenesis of idiopathic parkinsonism. Part 3: predicted probability and gradients of severity of idiopathic parkinsonism based on H. pylori antibody profile. *Helicobacter.* 2005;10:288-297.
120. de Luis DA, Varela C, de La Calle H, et al. Helicobacter pylori infection is markedly increased in patients with autoimmune atrophic thyroiditis. *J Clin Gastroenterol.* 1998;26:259-263.
121. Figura N, Di Cairano G, Lore F, et al. The infection by Helicobacter pylori strains expressing CagA is highly prevalent in women with autoimmune thyroid disorders. *J Physiol Pharmacol.* 1999;50:817-826.
122. Larizza D, Calcaterra V, Martinetti M, et al. Helicobacter pylori infection and autoimmune thyroid disease in young patients: the disadvantage of carrying the human leukocyte antigen-DRB1*0301 allele. *J Clin Endocrinol Metab.* 2006;91:176-179.
123. Franceschi F, Satta MA, Mentella MC, et al. Helicobacter pylori infection in patients with Hashimoto's thyroiditis. *Helicobacter.* 2004;9:369.
124. Sagaert X, De Wolf-Peeters C, Noels H, Baens M. The pathogenesis of MALT lymphomas: where do we stand? *Leukemia.* 2007;21:389-396.
125. Arima N, Tsudo M. Extragastric mucosa-associated lymphoid tissue lymphoma showing the regression by Helicobacter pylori eradication therapy. *Br J Haematol.* 2003;120:790-792.
126. Morinaka S, Tominaga M, Nakamura H. Detection of Helicobacter pylori in the middle ear fluid of patients with otitis media with effusion. *Otolaryngol Head Neck Surg.* 2005;133:791-794.
127. Szlachcic A. The link between Helicobacter pylori infection and rosacea. *J Eur Acad Dermatol Venereol.* 2002;16:328-333.
128. El Miedany YM, Baddour M, Ahmed I, Fahmy H. Sjogren's syndrome: concomitant H. pylori infection and possible correlation with clinical parameters. *Joint Bone Spine.* 2005;72:135-141.
129. Matysiak-Budnik T, Heyman M. Food allergy and Helicobacter pylori. *J Pediatr Gastroenterol Nutr.* 2002;34:5-12.
130. Rashid T, Ebringer A. Ankylosing spondylitis is linked to Klebsiella-the evidence. *Clin Rheumatol.* 2007;26:858-864.
131. Ebringer A, Rashid T, Tiwana H, Wilson C. A possible link between Crohn's disease and ankylosing spondylitis via Klebsiella infections. *Clin Rheumatol.* 2007;26:289-297.
132. Corapcioglu D, Tonyukuk V, Kiyan M, et al. Relationship between thyroid autoimmunity and Yersinia enterocolitica antibodies. *Thyroid.* 2002;12:613-617.
133. Leirisalo-Repo M, Hannu T, Mattila L. Microbial factors in spondyloarthropathies: insights from population studies. *Curr Opin Rheumatol.* 2003;15:408-412.
134. Douglas MR, Winer JB. Guillain-Barre syndrome and its treatment. *Expert Rev Neurother.* 2006;6:1569-1574.
135. Karch H, Tarr PI, Bielaszewska M. Enterohaemorrhagic Escherichia coli in human medicine. *Int J Med Microbiol.* 2005;295:405-418.
136. Faergemann J. Atopic dermatitis and fungi. *Clin Microbiol Rev.* 2002;15:545-563.
137. Bassi A, Dodd S, Williamson P, Bodger K. Cost of illness of inflammatory bowel disease in the UK: a single centre retrospective study. *Gut.* 2004;53:1471-1478.
138. Podolsky DK. Inflammatory bowel disease. *N Engl J Med.* 2002;347:417-429.
139. Hanauer SB. Inflammatory bowel disease: epidemiology, pathogenesis, and therapeutic opportunities. *Inflamm Bowel Dis.* 2006;12 Suppl 1:S3-9.
140. Das KM. Relationship of extraintestinal involvements in inflammatory bowel disease: new insights into autoimmune pathogenesis. *Dig Dis Sci.* 1999;44:1-13.
141. Kethu SR. Extraintestinal manifestations of inflammatory bowel diseases. *J Clin Gastroenterol.* 2006;40:467-475.
142. Loftus EV, Jr., Sandborn WJ. Epidemiology of inflammatory bowel disease. *Gastroenterol Clin North Am.* 2002;31:1-20.
143. Lakatos PL. Recent trends in the epidemiology of inflammatory bowel diseases: up or down? *World J Gastroenterol.* 2006;12:6102-6108.
144. Loftus EV, Jr. Clinical epidemiology of inflammatory bowel disease: Incidence, prevalence, and environmental influences. *Gastroenterology.* 2004;126:1504-1517.
145. Baumgart DC, Carding SR. Inflammatory bowel disease: cause and immunobiology. *Lancet.* 2007;369:1627-1640.
146. Phavichitr N, Cameron DJ, Catto-Smith AG. Increasing incidence of Crohn's disease in Victorian children. *J Gastroenterol Hepatol.* 2003;18:329-332.
147. Bouma G, Strober W. The immunological and genetic basis of inflammatory bowel disease. *Nat Rev Immunol.* 2003;3:521-533.
148. Danese S, Semeraro S, Papa A, et al. Extraintestinal manifestations in inflammatory bowel disease. *World J Gastroenterol.* 2005;11:7227-7236.
149. Evans PE, Pardi DS. Extraintestinal manifestations of inflammatory bowel disease: focus on the musculoskeletal, dermatologic, and ocular manifestations. *MedGenMed.* 2007;9:55.
150. Rothfuss KS, Stange EF, Herrlinger KR. Extraintestinal manifestations and complications in inflammatory bowel diseases. *World J Gastroenterol.* 2006;12:4819-4831.
151. De Vos M. Review article: joint involvement in inflammatory bowel disease. *Aliment Pharmacol Ther.* 2004;20 Suppl 4:36-42.
152. Schulte CM. Review article: bone disease in inflammatory bowel disease. *Aliment Pharmacol Ther.* 2004;20 Suppl 4:43-49.
153. Tavarela Veloso F. Review article: skin complications associated with inflammatory bowel disease. *Aliment Pharmacol Ther.* 2004;20 Suppl 4:50-53.
154. Itzkowitz SH, Harpaz N. Diagnosis and management of dysplasia in patients with inflammatory bowel diseases. *Gastroenterology.* 2004;126:1634-1648.
155. Itzkowitz SH, Yio X. Inflammation and cancer IV. Colorectal cancer in inflammatory bowel disease: the role of inflammation. *Am J Physiol Gastrointest Liver Physiol.* 2004;287:G7-17.
156. Bodger K. Cost of illness of Crohn's disease. *Pharmacoeconomics.* 2002;20:639-652.
157. Bernstein CN, Papineau N, Zajaczkowski J, Rawsthorne P, Okrusko G, Blanchard JF. Direct hospital costs for patients with inflammatory bowel disease in a Canadian tertiary care university hospital. *Am J Gastroenterol.* 2000;95:677-683.

158. Graff LA, Walker JR, Lix L, et al. The relationship of inflammatory bowel disease type and activity to psychological functioning and quality of life. *Clin Gastroenterol Hepatol.* 2006;4:1491-1501.
159. Irvine EJ. Review article: patients' fears and unmet needs in inflammatory bowel disease. *Aliment Pharmacol Ther.* 2004;20 Suppl 4:54-59.
160. Braun J, Sieper J. Building consensus on nomenclature and disease classification for ankylosing spondylitis: results and discussion of a questionnaire prepared for the International Workshop on New Treatment Strategies in Ankylosing Spondylitis, Berlin, Germany, 18-19 January 2002. *Ann Rheum Dis.* 2002;61 Suppl 3:iii61-67.
161. Sieper J, Braun J, Rudwaleit M, Boonen A, Zink A. Ankylosing spondylitis: an overview. *Ann Rheum Dis.* 2002;61 Suppl 3:iii8-18.
162. Sieper J, Rudwaleit M, Khan MA, Braun J. Concepts and epidemiology of spondyloarthritis. *Best Pract Res Clin Rheumatol.* 2006;20:401-417.
163. Rudwaleit M, Baeten D. Ankylosing spondylitis and bowel disease. *Best Pract Res Clin Rheumatol.* 2006;20:451-471.
164. Mau W, Zeidler H, Mau R, et al. Clinical features and prognosis of patients with possible ankylosing spondylitis. Results of a 10-year followup. *J Rheumatol.* 1988;15:1109-1114.
165. Braun J, Sieper J. Ankylosing spondylitis. *Lancet.* 2007;369:1379-1390.
166. Boonen A, van der Linden SM. The burden of ankylosing spondylitis. *J Rheumatol Suppl.* 2006;78:4-11.
167. Lawrence RC, Helmick CG, Arnett FC, et al. Estimates of the prevalence of arthritis and selected musculoskeletal disorders in the United States. *Arthritis Rheum.* 1998;41:778-799.
168. Mallbris L, Ritchlin CT, Stahle M. Metabolic disorders in patients with psoriasis and psoriatic arthritis. *Curr Rheumatol Rep.* 2006;8:355-363.
169. El Maghraoui A. Pleuropulmonary involvement in ankylosing spondylitis. *Joint Bone Spine.* 2005;72:496-502.
170. Banares A, Hernandez-Garcia C, Fernandez-Gutierrez B, Jover JA. Eye involvement in the spondyloarthropathies. *Rheum Dis Clin North Am.* 1998;24:771-784, ix.
171. Peters MJ, van der Horst-Bruinsma IE, Dijkmans BA, Nurmohamed MT. Cardiovascular risk profile of patients with spondylarthropathies, particularly ankylosing spondylitis and psoriatic arthritis. *Semin Arthritis Rheum.* 2004;34:585-592.
172. Greaves ML, Pochapin M. Asymptomatic ileitis: past, present, and future. *J Clin Gastroenterol.* 2006;40:281-285.
173. Ward MM. Health-related quality of life in ankylosing spondylitis: a survey of 175 patients. *Arthritis Care Res.* 1999;12:247-255.
174. Zhao LK, Liao ZT, Li CH, et al. Evaluation of quality of life using ASQoL questionnaire in patients with ankylosing spondylitis in a Chinese population. *Rheumatol Int.* 2007;27:605-611.
175. Kobelt G, Andlin-Sobocki P, Maksymowych WP. Costs and quality of life of patients with ankylosing spondylitis in Canada. *J Rheumatol.* 2006;33:289-295.
176. O'Byrne KJ, Dalgleish AG. Chronic immune activation and inflammation as the cause of malignancy. *Br J Cancer.* 2001;85:473-483.
177. Rao VP, Poutahidis T, Fox JG, Erdman SE. Breast cancer: should gastrointestinal bacteria be on our radar screen? *Cancer Res.* 2007;67:847-850.
178. American Cancer Society. Cancer Facts & Figures 2007. http://www.cancer.org/docroot/STT/content/STT_1x_Cancer_Facts__Figures_2007.asp. Accessed Feb. 12, 2008.
179. Jemal A, Siegel R, Ward E, Murray T, Xu J, Thun MJ. Cancer statistics, 2007. *CA Cancer J Clin.* 2007;57:43-66.
180. Chen X, Yang CS. Esophageal adenocarcinoma: a review and perspectives on the mechanism of carcinogenesis and chemoprevention. *Carcinogenesis.* 2001;22:1119-1129.
181. Lagergren J, Bergstrom R, Lindgren A, Nyren O. Symptomatic gastroesophageal reflux as a risk factor for esophageal adenocarcinoma. *N Engl J Med.* 1999;340:825-831.
182. Parkin DM, Bray F, Ferlay J, Pisani P. Global cancer statistics, 2002. *CA Cancer J Clin.* 2005;55:74-108.
183. Enzinger PC, Mayer RJ. Esophageal cancer. *N Engl J Med.* 2003;349:2241-2252.
184. Higaki S, Akazawa A, Nakamura H, Yanai H, Yoshida T, Okita K. Metaplastic polyp of the colon develops in response to inflammation. *J Gastroenterol Hepatol.* 1999;14:709-714.
185. Greenstein AJ, Mullin GE, Strauchen JA, et al. Lymphoma in inflammatory bowel disease. *Cancer.* 1992;69:1119-1123.
186. American Cancer Society. Costs of Cancer. http://www.cancer.org/docroot/MIT/content/MIT_3_2X_Costs_of_Cancer.asp. Accessed Feb. 12, 2008.
187. Meropol NJ, Schulman KA. Cost of cancer care: issues and implications. *J Clin Oncol.* 2007;25:180-186.
188. Kim P. Cost of cancer care: the patient perspective. *J Clin Oncol.* 2007;25:228-232.
189. Corazziari E. Definition and epidemiology of functional gastrointestinal disorders. *Best Pract Res Clin Gastroenterol.* 2004;18:613-631.
190. Drossman DA, Camilleri M, Mayer EA, Whitehead WE. AGA technical review on irritable bowel syndrome. *Gastroenterology.* 2002;123:2108-2131.
191. Drossman DA. The functional gastrointestinal disorders and the Rome II process. *Gut.* 1999;45 Suppl 2:II1-5.
192. Everhart JE, Renault PF. Irritable bowel syndrome in office-based practice in the United States. *Gastroenterology.* 1991;100:998-1005.
193. Drossman DA, Dumitrascu DL. Rome III: New standard for functional gastrointestinal disorders. *J Gastrointestin Liver Dis.* 2006;15:237-241.
194. Drossman DA. Irritable bowel syndrome: how far do you go in the workup? *Gastroenterology.* 2001;121:1512-1515.
195. Horwitz BJ, Fisher RS. The irritable bowel syndrome. *N Engl J Med.* 2001;344:1846-1850.
196. Evidence-based position statement on the management of irritable bowel syndrome in North America. *Am J Gastroenterol.* 2002;97:S1-5.
197. Koloski NA, Talley NJ, Boyce PM. Predictors of health care seeking for irritable bowel syndrome and nonulcer dyspepsia: a critical review of the literature on symptom and psychosocial factors. *Am J Gastroenterol.* 2001;96:1340-1349.
198. Cremonini F, Talley NJ. Irritable bowel syndrome: epidemiology, natural history, health care seeking and emerging risk factors. *Gastroenterol Clin North Am.* 2005;34:189-204.
199. Whitehead WE, Palsson O, Jones KR. Systematic review of the comorbidity of irritable bowel syndrome with other disorders: what are the causes and implications? *Gastroenterology.* 2002;122:1140-1156.
200. Cash B, Sullivan S, Barghout V. Total costs of IBS: employer and managed care perspective. *Am J Manag Care.* 2005;11:S7-16.
201. Goetzel RZ, Hawkins K, Ozminkowski RJ, Wang S. The health and productivity cost burden of the "top 10" physical and mental health conditions affecting six large U.S. employers in 1999. *J Occup Environ Med.* 2003;45:5-14.
202. Talley NJ, Zinsmeister AR, Melton LJ, 3rd. Irritable bowel syndrome in a community: symptom subgroups, risk factors, and health care utilization. *Am J Epidemiol.* 1995;142:76-83.
203. Dean BB, Aguilar D, Barghout V, et al. Impairment in work productivity and health-related quality of life in patients with IBS. *Am J Manag Care.* 2005;11:S17-26.
204. Frank L, Kleinman L, Rentz A, Ciesla G, Kim JJ, Zacker C. Health-related quality of life associated with irritable bowel syndrome: comparison with other chronic diseases. *Clin Ther.* 2002;24:675-689; discussion 674.

205. Talley NJ. A unifying hypothesis for the functional gastrointestinal disorders: really multiple diseases or one irritable gut? *Rev Gastroenterol Disord.* 2006;6:72-78.
206. Frissora CL, Koch KL. Symptom overlap and comorbidity of irritable bowel syndrome with other conditions. *Curr Gastroenterol Rep.* 2005;7:264-271.
207. Riordan SM, Kim R. Bacterial overgrowth as a cause of irritable bowel syndrome. *Curr Opin Gastroenterol.* 2006;22:669-673.
208. Spiller RC. Role of infection in irritable bowel syndrome. *J Gastroenterol.* 2007;42 Suppl 17:41-47.
209. Collins SM. The relationship of enteric microbial infection and functional bowel disorders. *J Clin Gastroenterol.* 2007;41 Suppl 1:S30-32.
210. Noureddin M, Lin HC. Role of Gut Bacteria in Patients With Irritable Bowel Syndrome. *J Clin Gastroenterol.* 2007;41 Suppl 1:S33-S36.
211. Kirsch R, Riddell RH. Histopathological alterations in irritable bowel syndrome. *Mod Pathol.* 2006;19:1638-1645.
212. Dunlop SP, Hebden J, Campbell E, et al. Abnormal intestinal permeability in subgroups of diarrhea-predominant irritable bowel syndromes. *Am J Gastroenterol.* 2006;101:1288-1294.

Chapter 2

Flora, Intestinal Permeability, and Immune Response

The idea that disruptions in gut function might be implicated in systemic disease is an ancient one. From an Ayurvedic text comes a definition of health as profound as any modern one: "A person whose basic emotional and physical tendencies are in balance, *whose digestive power is balanced, whose bodily tissues, elimination functions and activities are in balance*, and whose mind, senses and soul are filled with vitality, that person is said to be healthy (italics added)." In Hippocrates, we read the same idea, stated briefly as "bad digestion is the root of all evil."[1] The idea was further promoted in the 19th century by the naturopath Louis Kühne and in the early 20th century by Nobel laureate Elie Metchnikoff. Kühne proposed that an inappropriate diet led to intestinal toxicity, with increased growth of bacteria in the bowel causing disease. Metchnikoff believed that "death begins in the colon"; he held that many diseases were related to the action of gut bacteria and that consuming beneficial lactic acid-producing bacteria (in fermented milk) prevented growth of the putrefactive bacteria.[2] Although these pioneers did not use the word *inflammation*, the concept of intestinal inflammation is contained within their notion of intestinal toxicity.

In this chapter, we will discuss key concepts that are important to a modern understanding of gut inflammation and altered intestinal flora (dysbiosis) and their role in systemic disease. We will begin with a discussion of the structure and functions of gastrointestinal defense, focusing in particular on (1) the role of commensal gut microbes—the gut flora—in the development of a competent intestinal and systemic immune system and (2) the role of the epithelial intercellular tight junctions in maintaining a barrier between the intestinal lumen and the underlying immune system. We will then discuss how environmental factors and bacterial colonization (e.g., biofilms) may change the composition of gut flora and epithelial barrier function and how these changes may contribute to the pathogenesis and progression of disease. We also will briefly discuss the role of genetic factors in susceptibility to several diseases involving dysregulation of gastrointestinal flora and/or permeability, and we will update the hygiene hypothesis, which links modern changes in the composition of gut flora with immune dysregulation and disease. We will finish the chapter with specific examples of how alterations in gut flora and/or epithelial barrier function can lead to immune activation and thus to both systemic and local disease.

The story we will tell is one that begins in infancy, with the colonization of the gut by a variety of microbes, and that continues throughout the rest of life. It is incumbent on us as clinicians to understand this story. We must be able to identify what perturbs normal gastrointestinal function, to understand how those disturbances play out in the gastrointestinal tract and systemically, and to remediate the resulting dysfunction and disease. Genetics serves to identify individuals who are at greater risk for some of these debilitating conditions, but it is vital to remember that most genes do not represent a life sentence. They create a predisposition that may rest unexpressed until certain life events or environmental exposures tip the balance toward dysfunction.

Components and Functions of Gastrointestinal Defense

Components of Gastrointestinal Defense

A single layer of epithelial cells is all that separates the luminal environment, replete with antigens, from the vast array of immune regulatory tissue that lies directly beneath. There are in fact 3 essential components of the gastrointestinal defense mechanism[i]: gastrointestinal flora, the mucosal barrier itself, and the gut-associated lymphoid tissue (GALT). Balance among these 3 components is essential for effective protection from the potentially damaging external environment.[3]

Gastrointestinal flora — Bacteria are present in enormous quantities and with great diversity in the human intestine, including obligate anaerobes (gram-negative bacteria such as *Bacteroides* and *Fusobacterium*; gram-positive bacteria such as *Bifidobacterium*, *Lactobacillus*, and *Clostridium*; and gram-negative and gram-positive cocci) and facultative anaerobes such as *Escherichia coli*, *Citrobacter*, *Enterobacter*, *Proteus*, and *Klebsiella*.[4] In the stomach and small intestine, relatively low concentrations of bacteria are found (10^3–10^5 organisms per gram of luminal contents), but in the ileum, both the concentration and diversity of species increase. The distal part of the small intestine forms a transition zone, with bacterial counts increasing to 10^8 per gram. In the large intestine, concentrations of 10^{10}–10^{12} per gram are found; 90% to 95% are anaerobic. Bacterial species that predominate in stool, like *Bacteroides*, *Bifidobacterium*, and *Clostridium*,[5-7] are lumen dwellers. Bacteria that colonize the mucosal surface, predominantly spirochetes and fusiform bacteria, may not appear in stool.

GI Tract Site of Bacteria	Density of Bacteria	Common Bacterial Populations	
Esophagus		Lactobacilli	
Stomach	[10^3 – 10^5 /g]		
Small intestine			
Duodenum	[10^3 – 10^5 /g]	Lactobacilli Streptococci Enterobacteria *Bacteroides spp.*	
Jejunum	[10^3 – 10^5 /g]		
Ileum	[10^3 – 10^{12} /g]		
Large intestine	[10^{10} – 10^{12} /g]	*Bacteroides spp.* *Fusobacterium spp.* *E. Faecalis* Lactobacilli *Staph. Aureis* *Clostridium sp.*	Enterobacteria Klebsiella Eubacteria Bifidobacteria Streptococci Pseudomonas Salmonella
Feces	[10^9 – 10^{11} /g]	*Bacteroides spp.* Bifidobacteria Eubacteria	Coliforms *E. Faecalis*

Figure 2.1—Common Bacteria in the Gastrointestinal Tract

Reprinted from *Clinical Nutrition: A Functional Approach*.[8] ©2004, The Institute for Functional Medicine

[i] Physicochemical barriers are in actuality the first layer of defense against potential pathogens in the gastrointestinal tract; these defenses include antimicrobial peptides, mucins, trefoil peptides, and secretory IgA, all of which act to control the access of antigens to the underlying immune system. [Nagler-Anderson C. Man the barrier! Strategic defences in the intestinal mucosa. *Nat Rev Immunol.* 2001;1:59-67.]

Mucosal barrier — Mucus provides a structural layer of defense against pathogen invasion. Secreted by goblet cells, this substance is composed of mucin glycoproteins that form a gel-like film over the epithelial surface. [9, 10] Secretory IgA, produced by B cells in the underlying GALT and transported to the luminal surface of the gut epithelium, prevents both adhesion of antigens to the epithelium and interaction of antigens with the GALT.[11]

Junctions between epithelial cells constitute another important component of the barrier between the gut lumen and the GALT. These are known as tight junctions and are seen on electron microscopy to be discrete regions of cell membrane apposition at the apical junctions of epithelial cells. They serve to regulate the paracellular flow of solutes and fluid under normal circumstances and act as a barrier against the ingress of luminal contents and antigens.[12]

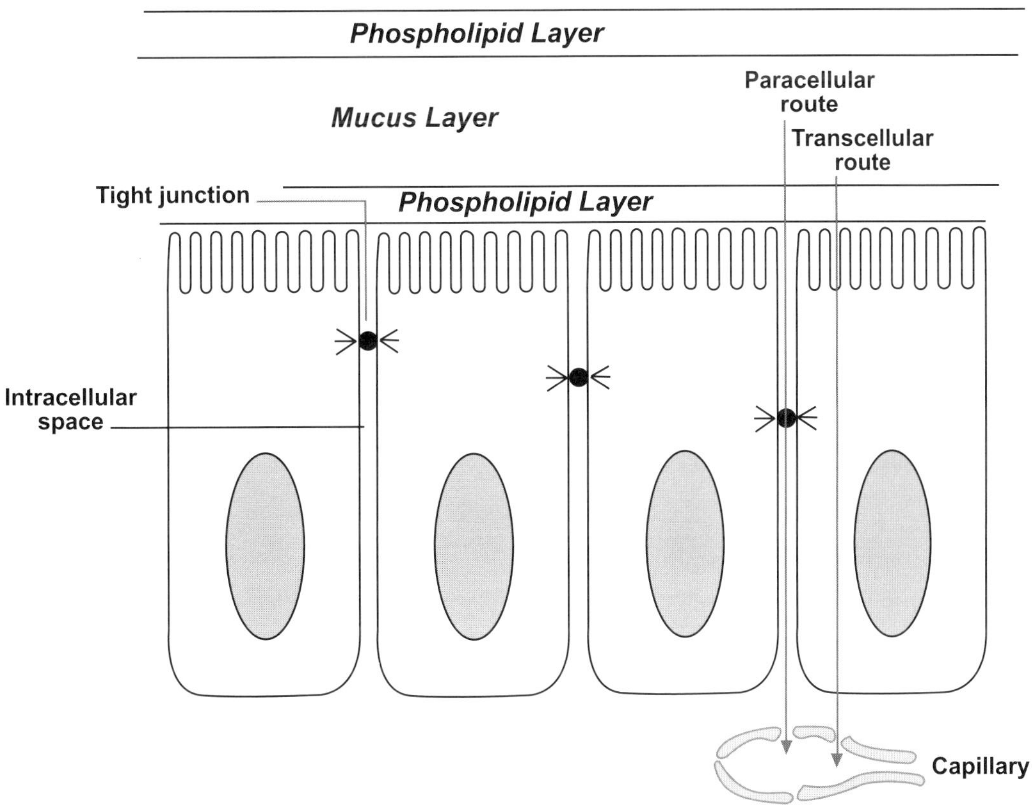

Figure 2.2—Epithelial Tight Junctions

Gut-associated lymphoid tissue — The GALT is the largest and most complex part of the body's immune system,[13] and more than 70% of the body's lymphocytes reside there.[7] Underneath the epithelial layer, with its mucus and tight junctions, the complex of immune tissue comprises both organized lymphoid tissue (in Peyer's patches and mesenteric lymph nodes), where induction of the immune response to antigen occurs, and cells scattered throughout both the epithelium and the lamina propria, which act as effectors of the immune response.[13]

Peyer's patches are macroscopic aggregates of lymphoid tissue, consisting of B and T cells, found along the length of the small intestine. Mesenteric lymph nodes are the largest lymph nodes in the body, distinct from Peyer's patches, and are thought to be the sites where interaction between local mucosal and systemic immune pathways takes place.[13] Peyer's patches are covered by a layer of follicle-associated epithelium, which is infiltrated by a large number of B and T cells, macrophages, and dendritic cells. Here the typical columnar epithelial cells of the small intestine are replaced by specialized M cells that bind and ingest particulate antigens. [9, 13, 14]

Functions of Gastrointestinal Defense

Gastrointestinal flora — Gut flora have a functional role in gastrointestinal defense, including protection of the intestinal epithelium from injury and maintenance of the architectural integrity of the epithelial surface through effects on proliferation and differentiation of epithelial cells. Mucosal microbes stimulate the secretion by epithelial cells of antimicrobial peptides[7]; they also cause an increase in the number of goblet cells in the gut epithelium, thus increasing mucus and trefoil peptide secretion.[ii] In addition, gut flora contribute to the induction of secretory IgA, which facilitates the sequestration of gut microbes to the luminal side of the gut epithelium.

Under normal circumstances, the gut flora do not trigger harmful inflammatory responses. Indeed, the development of immune tolerance to commensal bacteria is essential for normal immune function. In addition, commensal bacteria are essential to the development of *systemic* immune competence, at least in laboratory animals. Germ-free mice have been shown to have defective development of both spleen and secondary lymphoid tissue, as well as defects in the GALT.[15] (The lack of immune response to commensal flora is discussed in detail below.)

Commensal microbes in the gastrointestinal tract have several other important functions that are beneficial to the host.[3-5, 15-17]

- Competition with potential pathogens for space and resources
- Digestion of plant polysaccharides that would otherwise be unavailable to the host
- Promotion of monosaccharide absorption and triglyceride storage
- Synthesis of vitamins (K, B12, biotin, folic acid, pantothenate)
- Biotransformation of steroid hormones, bile acids, drugs, and dietary carcinogens
- Modulation of epithelial tight junctions and gut motility
- Production of n-butyrate as a fuel source for colonocytes

Mucosal barrier The tight junctions between epithelial cells form a selectively permeable barrier, with alterations in gastrointestinal permeability occurring in response to a variety of extracellular stimuli.[18] Several proteins, including claudins, occludins, and zonulin, appear to be involved in regulation of tight junctions, although their functions have not been fully elucidated.[12, 18, 19] Factors that affect permeability include pH,[20] melittin,[21] composition of the gut flora, food antigens, insulin, insulin-like growth factors, luminal glucose concentration, polyunsaturated fatty acids, nitric oxide, and cytokines.[22] Short-chain fatty acids[22] (by-products of starch metabolism in the gut) and prostaglandins[23] decrease permeability, and closure of tight junctions appears to be an important part of the repair of injured intestinal mucosa.[24] Enteric glia also appear to be involved in the regulation of tight junctions.[25] Disruption of the tight junctions may allow access by dietary or bacterial antigens to the underlying immune system, thereby potentially inducing disease and undermining immune tolerance. (See *Alterations in Gastrointestinal Permeability* below.)

Clinical Pearl:

Direct measurement of small intestinal permeability by the lactulose/mannitol challenge test is like measuring a sedimentation rate for the gut. Sequential measurements of intestinal permeability are an excellent way to gauge small bowel healing in patients with celiac disease, Crohn's disease, food allergy, or infectious enteritis.

Gut-associated lymphoid tissue — There are several ways by which antigens can gain access to the complex of immune tissue described above. M cells can deliver antigen to antigen-presenting cells in the subepithelial dome

[ii] Trefoil peptides are a family of small proteins expressed by goblet cells that are secreted onto the apical gastrointestinal mucosal surface. Their proposed functions include mucus stabilization, as well as stimulation and differentiation of epithelial cells during wound repair. [Familari M, Cook GA, Taupin DR, Maryatt G, Yeomans ND, Giraud AS. Trefoil peptides are early markers of gastrointestinal maturation in the rat. *Int J Dev Biol*. 1998;42:783-789. Ogata H, Podolsky DK. Trefoil peptide expression and secretion is regulated by neuropeptides and acetylcholine. *Am J Physiol*. 1997;273:G348-354.]

(the layer underneath the epithelium and just above the Peyer's patches).[9, 13] Dendritic cells in the lamina propria can take up antigen by "snorkeling," that is, putting out transepithelial dendrites into the gut lumen to directly sample antigens.[9, 11] And intestinal epithelial cells themselves appear to present antigen to the underlying GALT.

When potential pathogens move into the gastrointestinal tract, they bring with them pathogen-associated molecular patterns (PAMPs), highly conserved "generic" motifs that are abundant in microbes such as viruses, bacteria, and fungi. These broad molecular patterns (including lipopolysaccharides, lipoteichoic acids, flagellins, and viral RNA and DNA) are recognized by a variety of pattern-recognition receptors present on several cells on or close to the luminal surface of the intestine, including epithelial and endothelial cells, intraepithelial lymphocytes, subepithelial mesenchymal cells, macrophages, dendritic cells, fibroblasts, and adipocytes.[9, 26] These pattern-recognition receptors include cell surface toll-like receptors (TLRs) and cytoplasmic nucleotide-binding oligomerization domain (NOD) receptors such as NOD2, also known as CARD15.[7, 9] Several different TLRs have been identified, each recognizing different microbial motifs or patterns.[9] Stimulation of these pattern-recognition receptors initiates a signaling cascade that triggers activation of transcription factors (in particular nuclear factor-kappa B, or NF-κB), which leads to the production or activation of mediators of nonspecific immediate, or innate, cellular inflammatory immune responses. These mediators include neutrophils, proinflammatory cytokines, nitric oxide, prostaglandins, and leukotrienes.[3, 9, 14]

The arrival of antigen stimulates both innate and adaptive, or acquired, immune responses in the GALT. The adaptive immune response rests on balanced production in the mesenteric lymph nodes of specific cloned populations of T-helper cells. Under the influence of the cytokine secretion pattern of the antigen-presenting cells, naive T (Th0) cells will differentiate into Th1, Th2, Th3, or Th17 cells, each of which has different effects. Whatever their phenotype, these antigen-responsive primed T cells then leave the mesenteric lymph nodes via efferent lymph to travel through the bloodstream and the thoracic duct to the gut mucosa, where they induce local immune responses.[13]

Th1 cells are predominantly involved in cell-mediated immunity. Production of interleukin-12 by the antigen-presenting cell stimulates the production of IFN-γ, and the net effect on Th0 cells is promotion of differentiation into Th1 cells. The principal cytokines involved in the maturation and function of Th2 cells, on the other hand, are interleukin-4 and -5; Th2 cells prime B cells to produce antibodies. These 2 T-cell pathways cross-regulate each other's development and activity.[27] Although many scientists write about the T-helper cell lineage as if Th1 cells are proinflammatory and Th2 cells are anti-inflammatory (but pro-allergenic), the net effects of Th1 and Th2 activation, including the relationship of the cells to each other, are entirely dependent upon the biochemical milieu in which these cells act.

The discovery of Th3 cells, which primarily secrete transforming growth factor-beta (TGF-β) and are described as immune-suppressive T-helper cells, and of Th17 cells, which are cytotoxic T-helper cells, adds greater complexity to the present understanding of T-cell responses. Th3 cells were discovered through investigation of mechanisms involved in oral tolerance. Th0 to Th3 differentiation is encouraged by a milieu containing interleukin-4 along with interleukin-12 and TGF-β.[28] On the other hand, the combination of TGF-β with interleukin-6, a cytokine largely produced by macrophages, encourages the generation of Th17 cells (so named because they produce interleukin-17), which appear to play an important role in both antimicrobial defenses and autoimmune cellular damage.[29] The T-cell repertoire is therefore highly dynamic and changeable.

Even in the absence of pathogens, the gut and the GALT are constantly bombarded with antigens. For instance, a small amount of digested proteins are not completely broken down into their component amino acids and may be absorbed intact.[30] In the upper bowel, most antigen exposure comes from the diet; in the ileum and colon, the additional antigenic load of gut flora comes into play.[31] Under normal circumstances, the commensal bacteria residing in the gut lumen and food antigens arriving there do not trigger harmful inflammatory responses. Rather, they trigger an immune response whereby oral tolerance,[13] or "immune privilege,"[15] results. Products of gut flora and/or food proteins arrive in the subepithelial layer. Signaling by TLRs turns on the production of prostaglandin E_2 by the mesenchymal cells and macrophages and of anti-inflammatory cytokines such as TGF-β and interleukin-10 by the epithelial cells.[13] Under these conditions, the antigen is presented to naïve T cells in the mesenteric lymph nodes or

Peyer's patches.[9, 13] The T cells then differentiate into a variety of regulatory T cells, including $CD4^+CD25^+$ regulatory T cells, $CD8^+$ suppressor cells, T_R1 cells (which produce interleukin-10 and IFN-γ), and/or anti-inflammatory Th3 cells (which produce TGF-β). These specialized T cells act to damp down any potentially damaging inflammatory response in the gut. The antigen-presenting dendritic cells also interact with B and T cells in Peyer's patches or mesenteric lymph nodes to induce IgA production. B cells travel through the lymph and blood and return to the gut, where they secrete IgA that is transported across the epithelial layer and acts as a protective barrier against bacterial invasion.[7, 13] The immunological consequences of these complex but controlled processes are systemic tolerance and local immune homeostasis.[13, 15]

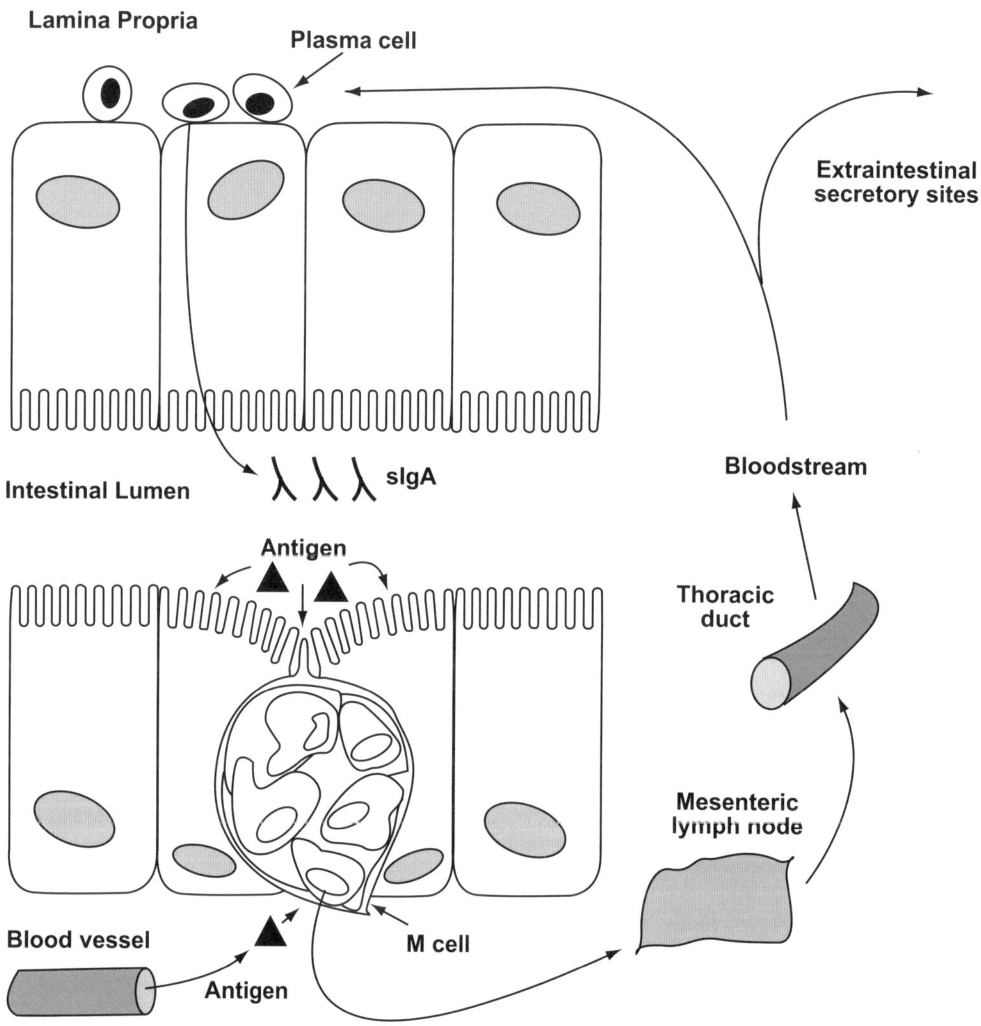

Figure 2.3—Development of Secretory IgA

Why gut flora do not trigger proinflammatory responses under normal conditions is not yet fully understood, since these bacteria contain patterns that are theoretically capable of binding to TLRs or intracellular receptors and triggering an inflammatory immune response in the same way pathogenic microbes do. It was noted as recently as 2005 that "it is

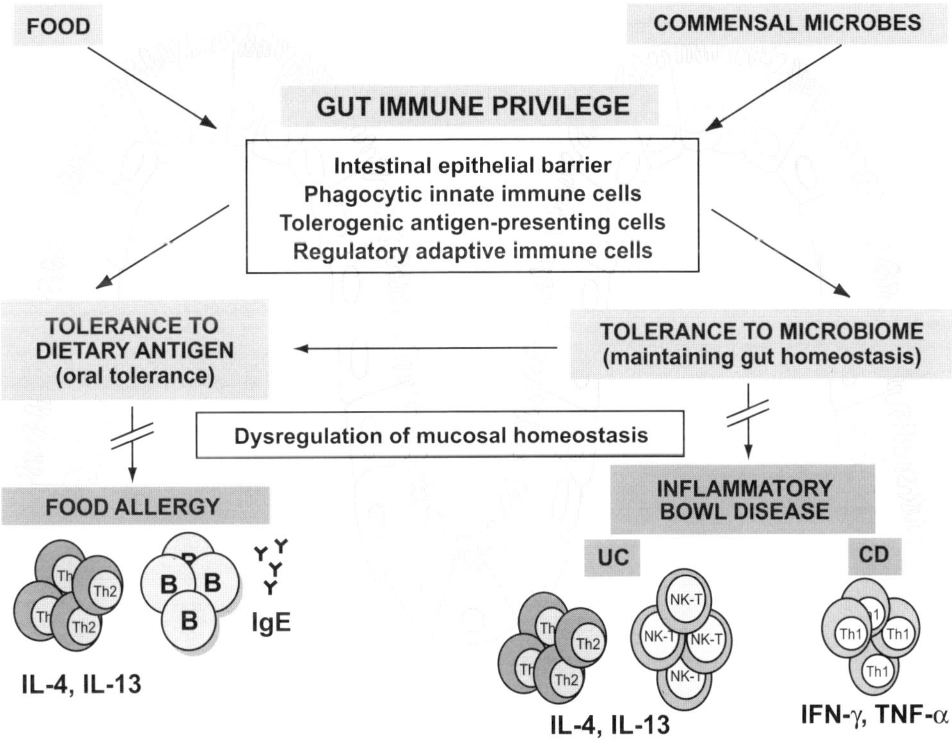

Figure 2.4—Development of Oral Tolerance

Immune privilege in the gut results from complex interactions between the gut flora, luminal dietary antigens, and the GALT. The different components of the GALT—the intestinal epithelial barrier, phagocytic innate immune cells, tolerogenic antigen-presenting cells, and regulatory cells of the adaptive immune system—integrate signals from intestinal luminal antigens to generate tolerance to dietary antigens and the maintenance of gut homeostasis. The tolerance of the gut to the commensal flora facilitates the establishment and maintenance of tolerance to foreign dietary antigen. In genetically predisposed individuals, disruption of tolerance to dietary antigens leads to Th2-mediated food allergies, characterized by increased production of IgE. Abrogation of tolerance to commensal microbes contributes to the development of inflammatory bowel disease. Reprinted with permission from *Immunol Rev*. 2006;213:82-100.[15] ©2006, Blackwell Munksgaard.

probably one of the most complex tasks to understand the mutual relationship between members of the microbial community in the gut and their interaction with the host."[32] The finding that serum from healthy humans contains antibodies to gut flora suggests that certain mechanisms modulate the immunity generated against commensal bacteria and promote immune privilege.[15] Mechanisms that may play a part in the lack of inflammatory response to commensal antigens [9, 13-15, 33] include:

- Inhibition of TLR signaling
- Presence of anergic macrophages
- Lack of expression of recognizable PAMPs by gut flora
- Differential expression of TLRs on epithelial cell surfaces
- Presence of suppressor lymphocytes and their associated cytokines
- Induction of regulatory T cells

Although M cells present particulate antigens to lymphocytes that show CD4 markers, and hence are immunogenic, columnar epithelial cells transport soluble gut-derived antigens and present them to CD8 lymphocytes, eliciting an immune suppressive response. To some extent, the balance between immune tolerance and immune stimulation in the small intestine may reflect the balance between these 2 pathways of antigen presentation.

The GALT response is connected to systemic immunity, and mesenteric lymph nodes play a central role in this connection.[13, 15] Mucosa-associated lymphoid tissue (MALT) -derived lymphocytes migrate to mesenteric lymph nodes and prime the nodal T cells, which then reach the systemic immune system and induce tolerance in response to intestinal antigens.[13] Nodal T cells also travel back to the intestinal mucosa, further modulating the local immune response. Gut-derived microbial antigens may also bypass MALT and mesenteric lymph node cells, gaining direct access to the systemic circulation, from which they may induce peripheral tolerogenic immune responses.[15]

To summarize, the GALT is extremely complex and involves interaction among microbes that are normal residents of the gastrointestinal tract, the junctions between gut epithelial cells that act as selectively permeable barriers, and the underlying immune cells. The system is designed to tolerate dietary antigens and certain friendly microbes, but also to recognize invading pathogens and to mount a vigorous defense when needed. The healthy gut makes such distinctions effectively, but dysregulation at any level in this system may have devastating consequences, not only for the gastrointestinal tract but for the organism as a whole.

Gastrointestinal Dysfunction: Causes of Dysbiosis and Increased Permeability

As a result of specialization within medicine that has occurred over the past 50 years, health practitioners have come to deal more and more exclusively with individual systems (the cardiovascular system, the respiratory system, the endocrine system, the liver, etc.), so that awareness of the role of the gastrointestinal tract in *systemic* health and disease has diminished. However, the high incidence of coronary artery disease,[34] certain cancers,[35, 36] atopic disorders,[37] inflammatory bowel diseases,[38] and other autoimmune diseases[39] has focused attention on the nutritional and environmental influences associated with these diseases. In particular, the recognition of the inflammatory nature of atherosclerotic disease[40] and cancer[41-44] has focused attention on inflammation as a cornerstone of many diseases of modernization.

There is currently no unifying theory regarding the role of gastrointestinal inflammation in these diseases. However, 2 key ideas have emerged that are related in terms of disease pathogenesis and, in particular, to the discussion above about immunologic and microbial homeostasis in the gastrointestinal tract. The first is the realization that *dysbiosis*, or disturbance in gut flora, may promote both local and systemic disease. The second is a hypothesis that *alterations in gastrointestinal permeability* may be involved in the pathogenesis of local and systemic disease. While both dysbiosis and alterations in gut permeability have always been relevant to local and systemic disease, it is only in recent years that our scientific understanding of these concepts and our ability to measure changes in gut flora and permeability have increased enough to make them accessible as clinical tools.

Dysbiosis

When the symbiotic nature of the relationship between gut flora and the host is disturbed, it can become injurious to the host, and organisms of relatively low intrinsic virulence, which had been coexisting peacefully with the host, may promote illness. This is termed *dysbiosis*, a term originally coined by Metchnikoff to describe alterations in gut bacteria resulting in a shift to more "pathogenic" bacteria in residence.[45] It is distinct from gastrointestinal infection, in which a highly virulent organism gains access to the gastrointestinal tract and infects the host. Since the commensal microbes in the gastrointestinal tract are critical for normal metabolic, trophic, and immune function in the gut, it is not difficult to understand how alterations in the composition or function of these organisms can have harmful effects.

There are several mechanisms by which alterations in the relationship between host and gut flora may predispose to gut inflammation and local or systemic disease,[3, 7, 18, 46-48] including autoimmune disease.

- Loss of commensal flora may allow overgrowth of pathogenic organisms that initiate local or systemic inflammation and disease.
- Dysbiosis may cause disruption of the epithelial tight junctions, with subsequent access of dietary or microbial antigens to both the underlying gastrointestinal immune system and to the systemic immune system.
- Dysbiosis may facilitate growth of microbes that directly damage the intestinal epithelial cells, exposing self-antigens which then initiate an immune response (this phenomenon is known as *bystander activation*).
- Components of gut microbial cell walls from pathogenic organisms may stimulate nonspecific, dysfunctional immune responses that produce local or systemic inflammation.
- Microbial antigens may cross-react with self-antigens and stimulate autoimmunity in a process known as *molecular mimicry*.
- Loss of certain commensal bacteria may facilitate failure of regulation of immune responses.

The principal factors that affect the composition and distribution of gut flora, as well as the interaction between gut flora and the host, are age, microbes, diet, drugs, and stress.

Age — The process of bacterial colonization of the previously sterile gut of newborns begins immediately after birth. The gut flora of babies comes to resemble that of adults by the age of 2 years,[49, 50] although Hopkins and colleagues observed that populations of facultative anaerobes in children were greater than those of healthy adults.[50] Colonization with beneficial bacteria is delayed in preterm infants and those born by cesarean section.[51]

The effects of age on gut flora have been summarized in several reviews.[49, 50, 52] Variations in fecal flora of infants tend to be large,[50] whereas in adulthood, the major bacterial groups in the feces remain relatively constant over time. In elderly patients, it appears that counts of total anaerobes and putatively protective *Lactobacillus* and *Bifidobacterium* species are decreased and that counts of *Enterobacter* and fungi are increased.[50, 52, 53] In addition, whereas *Bacteroides* species diversity increases with age, *Bifidobacterium* species diversity appears to decrease with age.[54] Increased populations of *Clostridium* species have been found in healthy elderly people.[50] Small bowel bacterial overgrowth is common in elderly patients and may be associated with malabsorption.[55]

Microbes — As would be expected from the profound effects of gut flora on the intestine and the immune response, the composition of gut flora has been shown to influence the susceptibility of the host to both gastrointestinal and systemic infection. Elderly patients who develop *Clostridium difficile*-associated diarrhea have decreased numbers of *Bacteroides*, *Prevotella*, and *Bifidobacterium* species.[54] In a recent animal study, mice with limited enteric flora were efficiently colonized at high levels with *Campylobacter jejuni*, whereas mice with normal enteric flora were colonized "inconsistently and inefficiently."[56] Small bowel bacterial overgrowth and increased bacterial translocation (migration of bacteria from the intestinal lumen to mesenteric lymph nodes or other extraintestinal sites) are both thought to be implicated in the increased potential for infection in patients with chronic liver disease.[57] The virulence of *Entamoeba histolytica* has been shown to vary depending on the composition of gut flora.[58]

Further evidence of the effect of gut microbial composition on susceptibility to infection is found in studies using probiotics, which are live microorganisms with potentially beneficial effects on the host. The research literature includes the following relevant studies:

- Manipulation of gut flora by administration of various species of *Lactobacillus* interfered with the pathogenesis of intestinal infectious agents such as *Rotavirus* and *E. coli*, although the exact mechanisms remain uncertain.[59]

- *In vitro, Lactobacillus* and *Bifidobacterium* species decreased infection with vesicular stomatitis virus.[60]
- In a meta-analysis of studies in which probiotics were administered to premature babies at risk of developing necrotizing enterocolitis (a common condition characterized by translocation of pathogenic bacteria across an intestinal wall with defective barrier function in the presence of abnormal gut flora), administration of probiotics resulted in a significant overall reduction in the incidence of necrotizing enterocolitis.[61]
- A recent meta-analysis of studies looking at the effects of probiotics on antibiotic-induced diarrhea and *C. difficile*-associated diarrhea showed that administration of *Saccharomyces boulardii, Lactobacillus rhamnosus* GG, and a probiotic mixture significantly reduced the development of antibiotic-associated diarrhea; in addition, administration of *S. boulardii* was effective in reducing recurrence of *C. difficile*-associated diarrhea.[62]

It must be noted, however, that in a recent trial of patients with predicted severe acute pancreatitis, probiotics did not reduce the risk of infectious complications but were associated with an increased risk of mortality.[63] (For more information on the effects of probiotics in specific diseases, see *Disease Manifestations of Dysbiosis and Permeability* below.)

There is also evidence to suggest that intestinal infection can have effects on gut flora. Decreases in *Lactobacillus* counts, for example, have been found in people infected with *E. histolytica*, including people with asymptomatic infection and with amebic liver disease.[64]

Clinical Pearl:

In administering probiotics, it is best to allow each patient to serve as his or her own control and track specific changes in symptoms or function over time. There is simply no "best" probiotic for any condition, whatever controlled studies may show, but there may be better probiotics for individual patients.

Diet — Commensal microbes are an integral part of the process of food digestion in the human gastrointestinal tract. Growth and function of gut flora are largely determined by the amount and type of substrate available from food ingested by the host.[65] Indeed, the gut microbial ecosystem should be viewed as a dynamic system that constantly interacts with food components.[66] What we eat, then, will influence the composition of gut flora.

Infant feeding practices can affect gut flora. It has been shown that breast milk contains *Bifidobacterium* species,[67] and breast-fed babies have higher fecal counts of *Bifidobacterium* species, whereas bacteria that may be associated with disease (e.g., *Clostridium, Bacteroides, Enterococcus, Enterobacter*) are rare. Formula-fed babies have more diverse microbial colonization; the development of a "bifidus" flora is unusual.[68] Facultative anaerobes attain higher cell densities in formula-fed babies.[68, 69] In addition, these babies have higher fecal concentrations of ammonia and other potentially damaging bacterial metabolites.[69]

It is well documented that specific dietary components may selectively stimulate growth of individual bacterial species in the large intestine. The most frequent studies in humans are those involving the use of *prebiotics*, which have been defined as "non-digestible food ingredients that beneficially affect the host by selectively stimulating the growth and/or activity of one of a limited number of beneficial bacteria in the colon."[70] Several studies in humans attest to the fact that consuming these nondigestible starches increases the growth of *Bifidobacterium* species, a phenomenon that has become known as the *bifidogenic effect.*[71] Substituting the fructans inulin or fructooligosaccharides (see Table 2.1 for a list of foods containing these starches) for dietary sucrose has been shown in humans to selectively increase fecal counts of *Bifidobacterium* species and to simultaneously decrease counts of potentially toxic pathogens such as *Bacteroides, Fusobacterium,* and *Clostridium.*[72] Also in humans, consumption of isomalt, a sweetener similar to sucrose but poorly absorbed in the upper gastrointestinal tract, increases fecal concentration of *Bifidobacterium* species.[73] Several other studies have found the same effect.[74-76]

Table 2.1—Prebiotic Foods[65, 71]

- Jerusalem artichokes
- Chicory
- Onions
- Garlic
- Leeks
- Bananas
- Tomatoes
- Spinach
- Oatmeal
- Barley
- Flaxseed
- Wheat
- Legumes

Several animal studies also provide evidence of the effect of prebiotics on the composition of gut flora. Feeding dogs a high-protein diet increased the fecal concentration of *Clostridium* species; feeding a diet high in nondigestible oligosaccharides, in contrast, increased concentrations of *Bifidobacterium* species.[77] In mice, consumption of a high-fat, low-fiber diet resulted in lower cecal concentrations of total bacteria as compared to mice fed a diet amended with inulin, a starch digested by probiotic bacteria; *Bifidobacterium* was detected only in the mice on the inulin-amended diet, whereas *Clostridium* and *Desulfovibrio* (a sulphur-reducing bacterium) were found only in mice on the high-fat diet.[78] Kleessen and colleagues fed rats a diet high in resistant starch (starches that are poorly degraded by pancreatic enzymes), which led to decreased cecal concentrations of *Bacteroides* and increased concentrations of *Lactobacillus* and *Bifidobacterium* species (as well as *Streptococcus* and *Enterobacter*).[79] Consumption of resistant starch by rats inoculated with human microflora has been shown to result in increased counts of *Lactobacillus* and *Bifidobacterium* species and decreased counts of *Enterobacter*.[80] In another study, pigs fed a diet high in inulin were more likely to harbor *Bifidobacterium* species.[81] Feeding rats a diet supplemented with fructooligosaccharides and inulin increased the concentration of mucosa-associated *Bifidobacterium* species.[82] In chickens, a whole-wheat diet significantly reduced the numbers of *Clostridium perfringens* in the intestinal tract.[83]

There is abundant evidence that other components of the diet affect the composition of gut flora.

- In one study, a vegan diet was associated with significantly decreased fecal counts of *Lactobacillus* and *Enterococcus* and somewhat decreased concentrations of *Clostridium* species; a lacto-vegetarian diet was also associated with somewhat lowered fecal concentrations of *Clostridium*.[84] In another study, Peltonen et al found significant changes in gut microbial composition (as measured by gas-liquid chromatography) after 1 month of treatment with an uncooked vegan diet, although the nature of the changes was not elaborated on.[85] And in a study of schoolchildren, an ovo-lacto-vegetarian diet was associated with decreased fecal concentrations of *Clostridium* and increased counts of *Bifidobacterium* species relative to children on an ad libitum diet.[86]
- A diet high in sulfur increases fecal counts of sulphur-reducing bacteria (principally *Desulfovibrio)*, which reduce sulfate and sulfites to sulfide[66]; sulfide is toxic to colonic epithelium.[65, 87] Sulfur is present in some preserved meats, dried fruits, and sun-dried tomatoes, as well as beer, wine, and cider.
- In another study, consumption of isoflavones (compounds found particularly in soy and flax products) led to marked changes in fecal bacteria composition, including increases in concentrations of *Lactobacillus* and *Bifidobacterium* species.[66]

- Although there does not appear to be direct evidence in humans of an effect of dietary fat on the concentration of *Clostridium* species in the feces, in a study of patients with gallstones (many of whom have a high dietary intake of fat), high concentrations of *Clostridium* were found in the feces.[88] *Clostridium* species can convert primary bile acids to secondary bile acids, which are carcinogenic[88-90]; it has recently been suggested, based on differing dietary patterns and colon cancer rates between Native Africans and African-Americans, that a high intake of animal fat and protein drives changes in the composition of the gut that ultimately lead to colon cancer.[91]

Consumption of certain foods may also affect the ability of pathogenic organisms to survive. Fermentation of Ghanaian maize dough resulted in decreased survival and proliferation of *Shigella* strains isolated from people with dysentery.[92] Whole-wheat feeding in broiler chickens that had been inoculated with *Salmonella typhimurium* decreased counts of the pathogen in the gizzard and ileum.[83] And administration of *S. boulardii* (in the form of a capsule) to school-children decreased the number of *E. coli* colonies in the feces.[93]

Liquid enteral diets have been associated with cecal bacterial overgrowth.[94] Tube feeding, known to be associated with an increased risk of *C. difficile*-associated diarrhea, has been shown to affect the composition of fecal flora, with a marked increase in the number of aerobic bacteria and a decrease in the number of anaerobic bacteria found in the feces of patients studied.[95]

Drugs — There are many drugs that affect gut flora, but we will start by discussing the most obvious—antibiotics. Antibiotic use[iii] is the most common and significant cause of major alterations in gut flora.[96] Changes in commensal bacteria increase susceptibility to infection by intestinal pathogens,[97] and overgrowth of already-present microbes such as *C. difficile* or fungi is a frequent cause of antibiotic-induced diarrhea, a well-known undesirable side effect of antibiotic use.[98] Factors that influence the effect of antibiotics on gut flora include the spectrum of activity of the antibiotic,[96] the rate of intestinal absorption, whether or not the antibiotic undergoes enterohepatic recirculation, and the dosage and length of administration.[99, 100] Antibiotics that are well absorbed in the small intestine have fewer effects on gut flora than poorly absorbed antibiotics. Enterohepatic recirculation increases the exposure of the gut to antibiotics and amplifies their effect.[98] Parenterally administered antibiotics can also recirculate in bile and therefore affect the composition of gut flora.[101] Broad-spectrum antibiotics, which have been increasingly prescribed, are likely to cause more severe disruptions in gut flora than narrow-spectrum drugs. Clearly, the greater the dose and the longer the dose is administered, the greater the impact on the composition of gut flora. The effects of antibiotics on gut flora can persist for days to months after administration stops. In one study, serum concentrations of enterolactone (produced via colonic conversion of plant lignins by gut flora) were reduced for up to 16 months after a single dose of antibiotics.[102] A full discussion of the specific effects of antibiotics on the composition of gut flora is beyond the scope of this monograph, but a 2004 review[103] provides detailed information on various antibiotics and their effects on the composition of gut flora; Table 2.2 summarizes research discussed in the review.

Although antibiotics are probably the most important drugs that affect the composition of gut flora, other drugs also contribute to the problem. Proton pump inhibitors, used to suppress gastric acid secretion, are in widespread use; there was a 10-fold increase in prescriptions in the United Kingdom between 1991 and 1995.[104] These drugs predispose the host (through the loss of gastric acid as a first-line defense against invasion by pathogens) to enteric infection with pathogenic organisms. Proton pump inhibitors also lead to the overgrowth of bacteria in the stomach and upper small intestine because of the change in pH, although the evidence that this overgrowth results in disease is not definitive.[105]

[iii] The problem of antibiotic resistance is well recognized and has been deemed a public health crisis in the United States. Indeed, the Centers for Disease Control and Prevention, along with other organizations such as the American Academy of Family Physicians and the American Academy of Pediatrics, have engaged for the past several years in a campaign to encourage more judicious prescribing of antibiotics. See *A Public Health Action Plan to Combat Antimicrobial Resistance.* Available online at http://www.cdc.gov/drugresistance/actionplan/. Accessed February 26, 2008.

Table 2.2—Effects of Selected Antibiotics on Gut Flora[103]

Agent	Impact on Enterobacteria	Impact on Enterococci	Impact on Anaerobic Bacteria	Overgrowth of Resistant Strains	Other Information
Ampicillin	↓↓	↓↓	↓↓	+	Decrease in lactobacilli and bifidus; ↑ in *Candida*; decrease in production of short-chain fatty acids
Amoxicillin	↓	↓	↓	+	↑ in *Candida*
Amoxicillin/ clavulanic acid	-	-	-	+	
Cefactor	-	-	-	+	7 days to normalization of flora; decrease in bifidus; ↑ in *C. difficile*
Ciprofloxacin	↓↓	↓↓	↓	-	7 days to normalization of flora; ↑ in yeast colonization; no effect on bifidus or clostridia
Clindamycin	-	↑	↓↓	+	14 days to normalization of flora; 10% of drug excreted in bile; decrease in production of short-chain fatty acids; decrease in bifidus and lactobacilli
Doxycycline	↓	↓	-	+	No effect on short-chain fatty acid production
Erythromycin	↓	↓	↓	+	No significant change in lactobacilli or bifidus; ↑ in yeast colonization; decrease in production of short-chain fatty acids
Metronidazole	-	-	-	-	No significant change in lactobacilli, yeasts, bifidus, or short-chain fatty acid production
Phenoxymethyl-penicillin	-	-	-	-	14 days to normalization of gut flora; no significant change in bifidus; larger doses decrease lactobacilli
Tetracycline	-	-	-	+	↑ in *Candida*; decrease in bifidus and lactobacilli
Tinidazole	-	-	-	-	No significant change in bifidus, lactobacilli, or short-chain fatty acids

Key: ↓↓ = strong suppression (>4 log 10 CFU/g feces); ↓ = mild to moderate suppression (2–4 log 10 CFU/g feces); ↑ = increase in number of organisms during therapy; - = no significant change; + = positive result

Drugs that affect gastrointestinal motility also affect the composition of gut flora.[17] Morphine has been shown to disrupt normal gut motility and result in small bowel bacterial overgrowth.[106] Several other drugs, including narcotics, phenothiazines, vincristine, and loperamide, have been shown to cause colonic pseudo-obstruction,[107] which may predispose to changes in composition of gut flora.[108] Similarly, any drugs that increase gut motility, such as erythromycin,[109] may cause changes in the composition of gut flora. Chronic alcohol consumption affects gut motility and has been shown to predispose to small bowel bacterial overgrowth. [110] Chronic constipation has been shown to lead to changes in the composition of gut flora, with decreased concentrations of *Bifidobacterium* and *Lactobacillus* species and increased concentrations of potentially pathogenic organisms.[111]

Stress — Stress has profound effects on gut function, inducing changes in gut permeability, mucin and ion secretion, composition of gut flora, and bacterial adherence.[112] In monkeys, separation of infants from their mothers was found to induce brief increases in *Lactobacillus* shedding on the first day, followed by a decrease in fecal concentration of *Lactobacillus* species and an increase in susceptibility to opportunistic infection.[113] Stress, in conjunction with starvation, has been shown to increase bacterial adherence to the mucosa in rats (along with increased permeability and decreased secretion of secretory IgA). These changes were attenuated with normal feeding.[114] Stress has also been shown to increase transcellular uptake of normally noninvasive luminal microbes by M cells in rats.[115] *In vitro* studies showed that catecholamines stimulate the growth of enteric bacteria such as commensal *E. coli* strains.[116, 117] In terms of the effects of stress on the composition of human gut flora, a study reported in 1976 found that *Bacteroides fragilis* in the feces was increased under stress and decreased to normal when the stressor was removed.[118] Another study, reported in 1987, found decreases in stool concentrations of *Lactobacillus* and *Bifidobacterium* species before space missions.[119]

Commensal microbes, then, are critical to well-being, but common experiences and exposures cause changes in the composition of gut flora that may have profound effects on the host, predisposing to and actually inducing both gastrointestinal and systemic disease.

Alterations in Gastrointestinal Permeability

We now turn to a discussion of several factors that are felt to disrupt gastrointestinal permeability, mainly by disturbing the integrity of the epithelial tight junctions. As we discussed earlier, maintenance of an appropriate barrier between the gut luminal contents and the GALT is essential in order to avoid continued interaction of the GALT with foreign antigens.

Age — The neonatal period represents a particularly challenging time in terms of gut permeability. In premature babies, permeability is increased in the first days of life as compared with full-term babies.[136, 137] Several factors are believed to affect permeability during the neonatal period, including the presence or absence of enteral feeding, the degree of acidosis, and the severity of intercurrent illness.[136] Beyond the neonatal period, permeability does not appear to increase with age under normal circumstances in either animals or humans,[138, 139] although the evidence is sparse.

Microbes — It is now known that the ability to alter epithelial tight junctions is a property of many infectious agents,[12, 18, 19] which can act directly to increase permeability, either by direct cleavage of tight junction proteins, by production of toxins that modulate permeability, or by expression of surface proteins that interact directly with E-cadherin (an epithelial cell adhesion molecule). Infectious agents also trigger innate immune responses, and the associated migration of polymorphonuclear cells may result in disturbance of the epithelial barrier.[19] Several infectious agents have been shown to increase permeability, and these are summarized in Table 2.3.

Table 2.3—Summary of Factors That Can Increase Gastrointestinal Permeability

- Infectious microbes[12, 18, 19, 120-125]
    - *Escherichia coli*
    - *Salmonella typhimurium*
    - *Clostridium perfringens*
    - *Bacteroides fragilis*
    - *Vibrio cholerae* (which has been shown to produce a peptide called zona occludens toxin, an analog of the physiological tight junction regulator zonulin)
    - *Entamoeba histolytica*
    - *Shigella*
    - *Listeria monocytogenes*
    - *Giardia lamblia*
    - *Clostridium difficile*
    - Influenza virus
    - Stomatitis virus
    - *Yersinia*
    - *Candida albicans*
    - *Trypanosoma brucei brucei*
    - Human immunodeficiency virus
    - *Rotavirus*
    - *Cryptosporidium*
    - *Helicobacter pylori*
- Food allergy[126]
- Iron supplementation[127, 128]
- Drugs[107, 129]
    - NSAIDs
    - Proton pump inhibitors
    - Platelet inhibitors
    - Antacids
    - Lipid-lowering agents
    - Mood stabilizers
    - Antidepressants
    - Potassium-binding resins
    - Chemotherapeutic agents
    - Corticosteroids
    - *Digitalis*
    - Diuretics
    - Oral contraceptives
    - Ergotamine
    - Methysergide
    - Pseudoephedrine
    - Sodium phosphate bowel preparations used to prepare patients for colonoscopy
- Alcohol[110]
- Stress[130, 131]
- Radiation therapy
- Thermal injury
- Circulatory compromise
- Hypoxia[19]
- Bilirubin[132-134]
- Total parenteral nutrition[135]

In contrast to the changes caused by pathogenic microbes, there is evidence to suggest that commensal microbes such as *Lactobacillus* may have beneficial effects on tight junctions and gut permeability. It has been demonstrated *in vitro* that *Lactobacillus* species can prevent aspirin-induced changes in tight junctions.[140] *Lactobacillus* species have also been shown to suppress stress-induced hyperpermeability in rats.[141] *In vitro*, the probiotic *E. coli* Nissle 1917 (used frequently in Central Europe to treat and prevent intestinal disorders) has been shown to abolish epithelial barrier disruption induced *in vitro* by enteropathogenic *E. coli* strains.[142] Research suggests that it may be the fermentation products of probiotics that act to maintain or improve tight junction integrity.[143, 144] In another animal study, colonic loops that had been stripped of normal flora were exposed to different bacteria. Colonization with *E. coli*, *Klebsiella pneumoniae*, and *Streptococcus viridans* increased absorption of mannitol, whereas colonization with *Lactobacillus brevis* reduced permeability to mannitol.[145] In experimental animals, both in the basal state and in conditions of inflammation such as acute gastroenteritis, intake of cow's milk supplemented with *Bifidobacterium breve* and *Streptococcus thermophilus* improved gut barrier function.[146] Mechanisms whereby commensal microbes may affect permeability include production of short-chain fatty acids, which may act directly on tight junctions through nutriture to the enterocyte,[147] and competition with other microbes known to increase permeability. This evidence confirms that many factors altering the composition of gut flora may also have detrimental effects on permeability.

Diet — Food allergy is known to be associated with increased gut permeability, which returns to normal after removal of the offending food.[126, 148] Most studies have concluded that increased permeability is the consequence, not the cause, of food allergy.[126] Environmental events such as enteric infections, ingestion of drugs, or stress may exacerbate the response by increasing permeability and facilitating the passage of foods across the gut epithelial barrier; the subsequent immune response may maintain a self-perpetuating cycle of antigen presentation and inflammation.[126]

In infants, it is unclear whether the type of feeding (breast milk or formula) affects gut permeability. In one study, permeability of infants was the same with a variety of different food preparations, including breast milk.[149] Another reviewer,[150] however, noted that several studies have demonstrated inhibitory effects of breast-feeding on bacterial translocation, suggesting beneficial effects on permeability. In an interesting recent study, significant amounts of endotoxin were found in a variety of infant formula preparations, raising concerns about their possible effects on permeability in formula-fed infants.[151]

Drugs — The list of drugs known to increase gut permeability is long. We concentrate first on nonsteroidal anti-inflammatory drugs (NSAIDs). It is ironic that these drugs, which have been effective at controlling musculoskeletal pain and inflammation for many patients, actually cause injury and ultimately intestinal inflammation in the gastrointestinal tract. The upper gastrointestinal problems associated with NSAID use have been well documented; these drugs are known to cause gastroduodenal ulcers and bleeding, which can be a major cause of morbidity and even mortality in NSAID users.[152] However, there are other, less appreciated, associations between NSAIDs, increases in permeability, and inflammation in the distal small intestine and large intestine.

NSAIDs are among the most prescribed drugs worldwide, particularly among older people. More than 30 million people worldwide use NSAIDs every day.[153] The toxic effects of NSAIDs can include several types of lesions that have been found in the distal small bowel, ranging from severe strictures and bleeding to a lower-grade "NSAID enteropathy" characterized by low-grade inflammation with accompanying blood and protein loss and subsequent hypoalbuminemia and iron-deficiency anemia.[154-157] These small bowel lesions have been found to occur in up to 75% of NSAID users.[155, 156] Enterohepatic circulation has been recognized as an important factor in intestinal injury by drugs, and it is now clear that continuous recirculation of NSAIDs and their metabolites increases delivery to the lower small intestine and increases damage.[98] Although the effects of NSAIDs on the large intestine are not as well characterized as the effects on the distal small bowel, NSAIDs have been found to cause large bowel pathology such as increases in complications related to diverticular disease, large bowel strictures, ulcers, and inflammation.[158-161]

The mechanisms of injury to the distal gastrointestinal tract appear to be at least in part independent of COX-mediated pathways.[162] It is postulated that 3 factors are responsible for the inflammatory and permeability changes seen in the distal small bowel and large bowel in NSAID users.

- NSAIDs (or their metabolites[98]) may interact with surface membrane phospholipids, leading to direct damage of enterocyte mitochondria.
- Mitochondrial damage leads to generation of free radicals, which cause increased permeability.
- Enterocyte damage and loss of normal barrier function leave gut mucosal cells and the underlying GALT vulnerable to interaction with luminal contents such as bile, food, bacteria (commensal and pathogenic), and enzymes, which results in inflammation.[155]

From a clinical perspective, it is important to note that this increase in gut permeability, which is similar in degree to that seen in people with Crohn's disease,[155] occurs within 12 hours of ingestion of a single dose of a nonselective NSAID and can persist after the drug has been stopped.[154] The associated inflammation may be detected even up to 3 years after NSAIDs have been stopped.[154]

There have been 2 case reports of small bowel enteropathy associated with low-dose aspirin therapy,[163, 164] although another study showed that fecal calprotectin levels (markers of inflammation) were not increased in a series of patients taking low-dose aspirin.[165] More than 36% of the American population, almost 87% of cardiovascular disease patients, and almost 63% of diabetes patients—over 50 million people—currently take low-dose aspirin for cardioprotection.[166, 167] Further studies will no doubt clarify whether low-dose aspirin is associated with increased gut permeability and/or enteropathy similar to that seen with NSAIDs.

NSAIDs are certainly not the only drugs known to be toxic to the gastrointestinal tract, and Table 2.3 provides a list of drugs, many of which are in common use, that can induce gastrointestinal inflammation.

Alcohol is associated with increases in gut permeability; alcohol intake has also been shown to cause transient endotoxemia both in healthy volunteers and in alcoholics with fatty livers. Furthermore, gut-derived bacterial toxins gaining access through increases in permeability associated with alcohol ingestion appear central to the development of progressive alcoholic liver injury.[110]

Stress — Several studies in animals[170-173] and a few in humans[130, 131] have shown that gut permeability is increased by stress, although the mechanisms remain incompletely elucidated. Mast cell activation,[131, 171] intestinal IgA depletion, corticotropin-releasing hormone release,[131, 172] nerve growth factors, cholinergic parasympathetic activation,[130] changes in secretion of ions and mucin, increased bacterial adherence, and permeability changes secondary to inflammation may all be involved.[112, 130, 131, 171, 172, 174, 175]

Because the immune system itself is involved in regulation of tight junctions, anything that induces an inflammatory response in the gut will affect gut permeability, whether or not it has a primary effect on tight junctions. It is not always possible to decipher whether substances toxic to the gut have primary effects on permeability or whether the noted alterations in permeability are secondary to an inflammatory response induced by direct toxic damage to the epithelial cells. Two proinflammatory cytokines in particular, IFN-γ and TNF-α, appear to have negative effects on tight junction integrity. These cytokines, which are found in high levels in intestinal mucosa in inflammatory bowel disease, have been found *in vitro* to decrease barrier function of intestinal epithelial cells.[18]

There is, then, a very important interplay between gut flora, epithelial tight junctions, and the immune system in maintaining gut (and systemic) health. Anything that disturbs any one of these three factors may induce changes in the other two, thereby contributing to disease initiation or progression (see Figure 2.5).

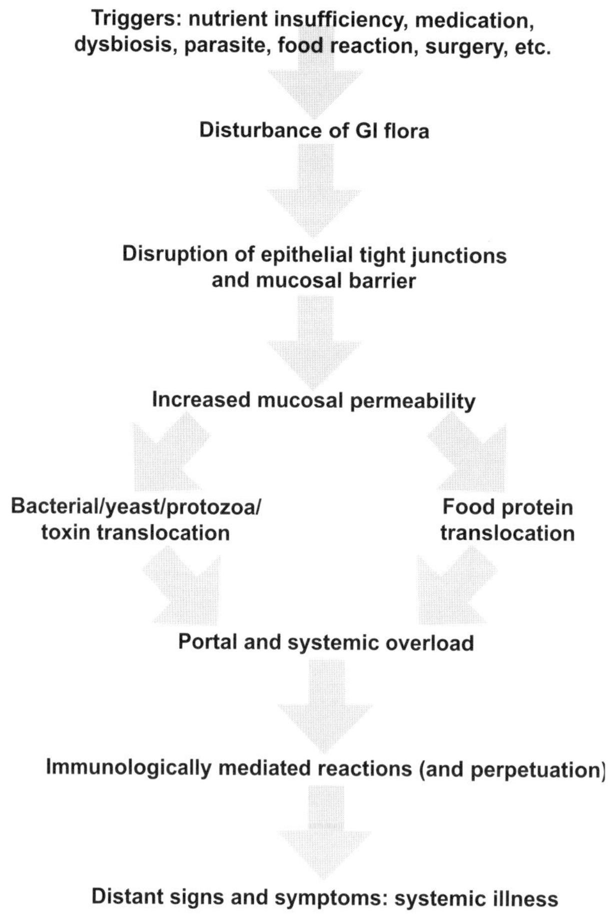

Figure 2.5—Factors in Gut and Systemic Health

Genetic Predisposition to Diseases Associated with Changes in Gastrointestinal Flora and Permeability

Certain diseases associated with disturbances of gastrointestinal flora and permeability, including autoimmune diseases, appear to have a genetic component; it is primarily the interaction between the genes and the environmental factors that produces dysfunction and disease. Three conditions are thought to be required for an autoimmune process to occur: (1) genetic susceptibility of the host immune system to recognize, and potentially misinterpret, an environmental antigen, such as bacteria, presented within the gastrointestinal tract, (2) exposure to triggering nonself-antigens, and (3) presentation of the antigen to the gastrointestinal mucosal immune system secondary to dysfunction of intercellular tight junctions. Therefore, gut permeability is a key factor in the development of disease, and the autoimmune response can theoretically be stopped and perhaps reversed if the interplay between the predisposing genes and the environmental triggers can be prevented or eliminated.[47]

Inappropriate reactions to gut microbes may also have a genetic component. For example, **ankylosing spondylitis** is a disease in which harmful immune interactions between gut microbes and the host[176] may be influenced by genetics. The association between the HLA-B27 gene and ankylosing spondylitis has been known for several decades; populations with a higher prevalence of HLA-B27 have a higher prevalence of ankylosing spondylitis.[177, 178] However, the fact that not all people with HLA-B27 develop ankylosing spondylitis—indeed, that most HLA-B27-positive people remain perfectly healthy[178]—suggests that environmental factors play a significant role in disease pathogenesis.

There are 4 theories to explain the function of HLA-B27 in susceptibility to ankylosing spondylitis:

- HLA-B27 may bind to an "arthritogenic" peptide (either bacterial or self), inducing a cytotoxic T-cell response.
- HLA-B27 heavy chains could unfold or change configuration, thereby inducing a proinflammatory response.
- HLA-B27-positive cells could kill infectious agents less efficiently.
- HLA-B27 could be recognized as autoantigenic because of its homology to a pathogenic bacterium.[179]

It has been suggested that molecular mimicry—the process whereby mimicry of host antigens by infectious agents may induce cross-reactive autoimmune responses which may tip the balance of immunological response and subsequently lead to autoimmune disease[180]—may be implicated in the pathogenesis of ankylosing spondylitis.[176] Amino acid sequence homology has been demonstrated between HLA-B27 and *Klebsiella* nitrogenase enzyme, between HLA-B27 and *Klebsiella* pullulanase enzyme, and between types I, III, and IV collagen and *Klebsiella* pullulanase enzyme.[181-183] Patients with ankylosing spondylitis have elevated antibodies to *Klebsiella* antigens, and serum from patients with ankylosing spondylitis is cytotoxic to cells coated with the HLA-B27 peptide homologous to the *Klebsiella* nitrogenase enzyme.[184] In addition, antigens expressing cross-reactivity between HLA-B27 and *Klebsiella* nitrogenase enzyme have been found to be strongly expressed in inflamed synovial tissue of patients with ankylosing spondylitis.[185] These findings have led some authors to suggest that antibodies to *Klebsiella* bind to cross-reactive antigens, triggering a cascade of inflammatory responses that eventually results in the clinical picture of ankylosing spondylitis.[176] Whether gut permeability is increased in ankylosing spondylitis patients is uncertain.[186-190]

Celiac disease is another condition in which genetic predisposition,[191] increased gut permeability,[47] and gut microbes[192-194]—as well as gliadin—may all interact to produce disease. It has long been recognized that the HLA-DQA1 and HLA-DQB1 genes are involved in the pathogenesis of celiac disease.[191] More recently, the MYO9B gene was also implicated.[191] MYO9B carries with it a Rho GTPase activation protein that regulates activity of the Rho GTPase enzymes, which are involved in regulating tight junction assembly, and it has been suggested that a genetically induced overactivity of the RhoA enzyme family increases permeability and facilitates the development of disease.[191]

Crohn's disease is yet another disease in which interactions between known genetic factors, gut microbes,[195-197] and gut hyperpermeability produce disease.[198, 199] Just as with ankylosing spondylitis, NOD2 (CARD15) has been identified as a susceptibility gene for Crohn's disease.[200] NOD2 is an intracellular signaling protein that, along with TLRs, plays an important role in both innate and acquired immunity as a sensor of bacterial components. In human gut tissue, the protein is expressed mainly in Paneth cells in the crypts of the terminal ileum.[201] Several mutations have been identified within the NOD2 gene. Exactly how these mutations result in disease susceptibility is not fully understood, and somewhat conflicting theories, summarized in a recent review,[200] have been proposed to explain the functional consequences of the observed NOD mutations.

- Because defective NOD2 signaling leads to defective activation of NF-κB, one theory is that this results in defective NF-κB-dependent Th1 responses and increased susceptibility to infection.
- Another theory is that defective NOD2 function results in defective epithelial cell function, with decreased secretion of antimicrobial α-defensins and increased susceptibility to bacterial infection.
- A third theory is that defective NOD2 function results in a failure of inhibition of signals delivered by TLRs, with subsequent enhancement of cytokine production by activated antigen-presenting cells.

The relative risk of developing Crohn's disease increases with the number of mutations. The fact that fewer than 10% of people with these polymorphisms go on to develop disease suggests that both other genetic polymorphisms and environmental stimuli are needed for disease expression.[200, 202, 203]

There is evidence to suggest that alterations in gut flora, combined with genetic susceptibility, play a role in the development of **atopic disorders**. The role of genetic susceptibility in atopy is complex and poorly understood.

Several genetic polymorphisms have been found in association with atopic disorders, but genetic heterogeneity across populations, the large variability in disease expression, and the presence of so many clinical disease markers have complicated the task of assessing the effect of genetic predisposition.[37, 204] Several genes have been identified as candidate genes in asthma, including C5 (complement factor 5), ADAM33 (expressed on smooth muscle and fibroblasts and involved in remodeling of the asthmatic lung), and DPP10 and PHF11, which are involved in cytokine and T-cell regulation.[204] Similarly, several candidate genes have been identified for atopic dermatitis (also known as eczema); interestingly, these genes do not overlap with the genes identified in association with asthma, but they do overlap with those identified for psoriasis and other skin diseases.[205] The fact that several of the genes identified for both asthma and atopic dermatitis are expressed in the mucosa and epidermis suggests that events at the epithelial surfaces drive the disease processes, focusing interest on mechanisms of innate immunity in disease pathogenesis.[206]

The Hygiene Hypothesis

We discuss here a particular hypothesis relating to the role of gut flora in the development of both atopic disorders and Crohn's disease. Crohn's disease is believed to be driven by Th1 cells, whereas atopic disorders are believed to be driven by Th2 cells. The hygiene hypothesis attempts to explain the role of the gut in the etiology of both disorders, even though they appear to have different pathogenetic mechanisms.

First published in 1989, the original hygiene hypothesis suggested that our modern hygienic lifestyle was predisposing us to develop allergic disorders because of decreased exposure to childhood infections.[207] Lack of exposure during childhood to microbes that would drive the activity of Th1 cells, thereby balancing the activity of Th2 cells, was postulated as an important factor in the rising incidence of atopic disorders.[48] Since then, however, it became apparent that there has also been a large increase in the incidence of several other diseases with deficient immunoregulation such as type 1 diabetes, Crohn's disease, and multiple sclerosis, all of which are primarily driven by Th1 cells. In fact, the incidence of atopic disorders (Th2 driven) and type 1 diabetes (Th1 driven) appears to correlate closely both within and outside Europe.[208]

The current thinking on the hygiene hypothesis, renamed the "microflora hypothesis" by some,[209] focuses less on exposure to infections and more on changes in the composition of gut flora and the role of these changes in diseases involving disorders of immunoregulation such as those mentioned above.[48, 210] Rather than focusing on the overactivity of Th1 or Th2 cells, the current focus is more on deficient activity of regulatory T cells, which modulate the activity of both Th1 and Th2 cells. This unifying theory provides a satisfactory explanation for the simultaneous rise in the incidence of diseases involving dysregulation of Th1 and Th2 cells.

The hypothesis has now been reworked to suggest that the induction of regulatory pathways involved in mucosal immunity occurs primarily in the GALT and that commensal bacteria are essential to that process. Changes in the composition of gut flora, and specifically the absence of certain protective bacteria, impair immune homeostasis and lead to allergic or autoimmune disease.[48] Support for this hypothesis comes from:

- Data showing defects in regulatory T cells in several diseases with increasing incidence (multiple sclerosis,[211] type 1 diabetes,[212] and allergic disorders[213])
- Changes in gut flora seen in patients with Crohn's disease[195-197] and atopic disorders[214-216]
- Data showing that probiotics can induce regulatory T cells in animal studies[217]
- Evidence that probiotics may be useful in the treatment of both inflammatory bowel disease[218] and atopic diseases[219]

In particular, there is increasing evidence that carriage of helminths, which are common residents of the intestine in the developing world but are being eliminated in Western societies, may protect the host from certain immunological disorders. Helminths appear to be protective against both Th1-driven disorders such as inflammatory bowel disease[220, 221] and the Th2-driven atopic disorders,[222-224] and the key protective mechanism in both diseases appears to involve the induction of regulatory T cells by helminths.[225, 226] Saprophytic *Mycobacterium*, *Bifidobacterium*, and *Lactobacillus* species are organisms that also induce immunoregulatory mechanisms in the host but that are now less frequent or even absent in the human environment of Westernized societies.[48] Several studies (discussed in detail below) have demonstrated the therapeutic effect of administration of probiotics such as *Lactobacillus* species in patients with atopic disease; these results speak to the therapeutic potential of probiotic agents in the multiplicity of diseases in which imbalanced gut flora has been implicated.

To summarize this section on causes of dysbiosis and increased intestinal permeability:

- Several factors relevant to modern life, such as diet, drugs, and stress, may alter the composition of gut flora, reducing its protective functions and thereby predisposing to disease.
- These same factors may also increase the permeability of the epithelial tight junctions, thus predisposing to disease by allowing interaction between microbial or dietary antigens and the underlying immune system.
- Certain diseases associated with changes in gut flora or permeability, such as ankylosing spondylitis, celiac disease, and Crohn's disease, also have a genetic component.
- The hygiene hypothesis suggests that modern changes in the composition of gut flora predispose to a variety of systemic diseases by changing the interactions occurring between gut flora and the gut immune system.

Disease Manifestations of Dysbiosis, Permeability, and Immune Dysregulation

In this section, we will explore the impact that alterations in gastrointestinal flora, permeability, immune response, and inflammation can have on patients vis-à-vis the pathogenesis of complex, chronic diseases, including both atopic conditions and autoimmune diseases. We have already discussed several autoimmune diseases in which gut inflammation is implicated, including celiac disease, ankylosing spondylitis, and inflammatory bowel disease. There is ongoing research into the possibility that changes in the composition of gut flora, changes in gut permeability, or abnormal immune responses to normal components of gut flora—all of which may result in gut inflammation—are implicated in the pathogenesis of several other autoimmune diseases such as atopic disorders, multiple sclerosis,[227] psoriasis,[228] systemic sclerosis,[229] IgA nephropathy[230] (an interesting study found an increased risk of celiac disease in patients with IgA nephropathy[231]), primary biliary cirrhosis,[232] rheumatoid arthritis,[233] and type 1 diabetes.[234, 235] Here we will highlight a few of these disorders. (For more information on the pathogenesis of rheumatoid arthritis and inflammatory bowel disease, see Chapter 4, *Antecedents, Triggers and Mediators: A Functional Approach*.)

Atopic Disorders

The term atopy (from the Greek *atopos*, meaning out of place) is used to describe diseases that are IgE mediated, including allergic rhinitis (hay fever), asthma, and atopic dermatitis.[37, 236] The newest nomenclature describes atopy as "a personal or familial tendency to produce IgE antibodies in response to low doses of allergens, usually proteins, and to develop typical symptoms such as asthma, rhinoconjunctivitis, or atopic eczema/dermatitis."[237] The atopic diseases are among the most common causes of chronic ill health, especially in children, and atopic diseases are becoming increasingly common in the Western world. In a study of the worldwide prevalence of atopic diseases among children aged 13 to 14 years, rates as high as 20% were found in several countries, including the United Kingdom, Ireland, Australia, and New Zealand,[236] and evidence suggests that the prevalence is increasing.[238] In Sweden, the number of children with atopic disease doubled between 1979 and 1991.[37, 236] The increase in the incidence of asthma has been termed an epidemic.[239] And allergic rhinitis, a disease that on the surface appears to be relatively minor and unimportant, affects between 20 and 40 million people in the United States.[238]

Dysbiosis — Although, as noted above, multiple environmental and genetic factors are probably involved in the pathogenesis of atopic diseases, the composition of gut flora appears to be a central factor; in particular, it appears that the absence of certain gut microbes predisposes to the development of atopic disease.[240] Differences in the composition of gut flora have been demonstrated between children suffering from atopic dermatitis and controls. Bjorksten and colleagues found that children with atopic dermatitis had decreased counts of *Lactobacillus* and *Bacteroides* species and increased counts of aerobic species, in particular coliforms and *Staphylococcus aureus*.[214] Distinct patterns of colonization of the gastrointestinal tract (present before the onset of clinical disease) have been documented in children predisposed to atopy.[214, 215, 240] The reasons for these patterns are unclear but may include different feeding practices, as well as changes in the vaginal flora of mothers.[240] In a study from Sweden, children raised according to the precepts of Rudolph Steiner's anthroposophical philosophy were less likely to develop allergic diseases than children raised in conventional families. Their quantitative stool cultures showed increased concentrations of *Enterococcus* and lactic acid bacteria compared to the control group.[241] Emerging evidence suggesting that probiotics may have a beneficial effect both on atopic symptoms in children and in primary prevention of atopic disease provides further evidence of a link between gut flora and atopy.[219]

Administration of *Lactobacillus rhamnosus* 19070-2 and *Lactobacillus reuteri* DSM 122460 for 6 weeks to children with atopic dermatitis resulted in improvement in symptoms in 56% of patients (15% with placebo), particularly in patients with positive skin prick test and elevated IgE levels.[242] In infants demonstrating atopic eczema during exclusive breast-feeding, weaning to an extensively hydrolyzed whey formula supplemented with *Bifidobacterium lactis* Bb-12 or *Lactobacillus* strain GG resulted in significant improvement in eczema, as well as a decrease in the concentration of soluble CD4 in serum and eosinophilic protein X in urine when compared with infants weaned to the formula unsupplemented with probiotics.[243] Probiotics have also been shown to benefit patients with allergic rhinitis. In one study, treatment of patients with allergic rhinitis with *Bacillus clausii* resulted in significant reduction in the nasal total symptoms score when compared with controls and was associated with a concomitant reduction in the nasal eosinophils count and the number of days of treatment with antihistamine.[244] In a recent study in which children with allergic rhinitis and/or asthma were given fermented milk containing *Lactobacillus casei* for a period of 12 months, the number of episodes of allergic rhinitis decreased when compared with the non-intervention group; no difference between intervention and control groups occurred in asthmatic children.[245]

A few studies have also examined the role of probiotics in the prevention of atopic diseases. Oral colonization 3 times in the first week of life in infants (not selected for family history of atopic disease) with a nonpathogenic *E. coli* strain (serotype 083:K24:H31) significantly reduced the occurrence of allergies (including rhinitis, asthma, and eczema) over a 20-year period when compared with the controls (infants not colonized with *E. coli*).[246] In another double-blind controlled trial, administration of *Lactobacillus rhamnosus* strain GG for 4 weeks prenatally to mothers with a family history of atopic disease, and for 3 months after birth to their infants, resulted in significant decrease in the frequency of chronic relapsing atopic eczema up to age 2 years in the treated group when compared with the placebo group. In addition, the concentration of (anti-inflammatory) TGF-β2 was significantly increased in the breast milk of the mothers treated with probiotics.[247]

Permeability — Alterations in gut permeability may also play a part in atopic disease; studies have demonstrated increases in permeability in both adults[248] and children[249] with asthma and in children with atopic dermatitis.[250] Administration of probiotics has been found both to reduce the extent of eczema and to decrease permeability.[242, 251]

Immune dysregulation — In an attempt to clarify further the role of gut flora in the development of the immune system and on the development of atopic disease, a large clinical trial, designed to assess the composition of gut flora, cytokine profiles, and development of atopy at 2 years, is under way.[252]

Rheumatoid Arthritis

Dysbiosis — Alterations in gut flora have been found in association with rheumatoid arthritis, although it is unclear whether these changes are involved in disease pathogenesis. An increased quantity of fecal anaerobic bacteria (measured by gas-liquid chromatographic analysis of bacterial cellular fatty acids in stool) has been demonstrated in patients with early disease, in particular those with erosive arthritis.[233] Higher fecal counts of *C. perfringens* have been found in association with active disease.[253] And macrophages and dendritic cells from the synovial tissue of rheumatoid arthritis patients were found to react with an antibody to gut-derived bacterial antigen.[254]

Permeability — There is evidence to suggest that alterations in gut permeability, with subsequent immune reactions to microbial and/or food antigens, may be involved in disease progression in rheumatoid arthritis, though not necessarily involved in initiation of the disease. There have been few studies assessing permeability in rheumatoid arthritis, but in those that have been published, permeability appears to be increased only in patients being treated (either with aspirin or other NSAIDs) and in patients with active (and therefore *presumably* treated) disease.[255-257] The connection between increased permeability and NSAID use in rheumatoid arthritis patients was noted in the 1980s,[258] and it was suggested at the time that although increased permeability might not be a primary factor in rheumatoid arthritis, NSAID use could contribute to increased presentation of dietary or bacterial antigens to the gut and systemic immune systems, thereby perhaps contributing to progression of the disease. [258] A British research group found that patients with rheumatoid arthritis had elevated IgA and IgG antibodies to *C. perfringens* toxin A and attributed the increase to the effects of NSAIDs, although permeability was not directly measured.[259]

Immune dysregulation — Evidence suggesting that exposure to gut-derived bacterial antigens is involved in the persistence or progression of rheumatoid arthritis comes from several studies demonstrating antibodies in sera, synovial tissue, and jejunal fluid of rheumatoid arthritis patients[254, 260-262] In a 2001 review, Toivanen[263] used the model of reactive arthritis to develop a model of rheumatoid arthritis pathogenesis. Noting that the cell walls of several microbes normally resident in the human intestine have been shown to induce proinflammatory cytokine production in mononuclear cells and that these cell walls can induce chronic arthritis in rats, the author suggested that bacterial cell wall peptidoglycans of normal microbial residents of the human intestine may, in genetically predisposed individuals, be the arthritogenic peptides responsible for rheumatoid arthritis.[263] Supporting evidence is provided by the finding that tetracyclines, in particular minocycline, are effective in the treatment of rheumatoid arthritis.[264] Although tetracyclines have other immunomodulatory effects in addition to their antibacterial properties,[265] it has been suggested that minocycline exerts its effect by modifying the composition of gut flora.[266] Further studies are clearly needed in order to clarify the role of gut-derived microbial antigens in disease initiation or progression.

Several studies examining the effects of different dietary modifications on symptoms and indicators of disease activity provide evidence that dietary antigens (rather than or in addition to microbial antigens) are involved in the persistence or progression of rheumatoid arthritis. A vegan diet free of gluten has been found to improve signs and symptoms of rheumatoid arthritis.[267] The mechanism is uncertain but is believed to involve reduction in presentation of dietary antigens to the immune system (as evidenced by the reduction in antibodies to food antigens shown in this study) or a change in the composition of gut flora, as has been demonstrated in other studies.[268-270] In another study, increased levels of antibodies to several dietary antigens were found in the jejunal fluid of rheumatoid arthritis patients.[271] In a 2007 study providing further evidence, an elemental diet devoid of whole proteins followed for 2 weeks was as effective as a course of oral prednisolone in improving subjective clinical parameters.[272] The authors suggested that the reduced antigenic load decreases immune activity in the gut mucosa, thereby reducing systemic inflammatory responses; decreased permeability is probably another factor.

Clinical Pearl:

There is no single diet that is best for patients with rheumatoid arthritis, but there are three types of diets that have shown beneficial effects in clinical studies: (1) a basic, nutrient-dense, high-omega-3, phytonutrient-rich, low-glycemic-index, anti-inflammatory diet, (2) an individualized allergy elimination diet, and (3) a gluten-free vegetarian diet. In treating patients with rheumatoid arthritis, I usually start with the basic diet and move on to the others based on clinical response and the patient's readiness.

Rheumatoid arthritis is one disorder in which fasting actually decreases intestinal permeability; presumably this is due to the removal of food allergens involved in disease pathogenesis.[273]

Crohn's Disease

Dysbiosis — Commensal microbes appear to play a central role in the development of Crohn's disease. Mutant strains of germ-free mice do not develop gut inflammation, but inflammation develops rapidly when the mice are colonized with commensal bacteria.[195] In humans, high counts of epithelium-associated *E. coli*, reductions in gut microbial species diversity, and dense adherent biofilms composed mainly of *Bacteroides* have been found in Crohn's disease patients.[196,197]

Permeability — Gut permeability is increased in Crohn's disease[198] (and ulcerative colitis[274]). As described in a recent review,[274] a reduction in tight junction strands, strand breaks, and alteration of tight junction protein content and composition characterize Crohn's disease; Th1 cytokine effects by IFN-γ and TNF-α are key factors in the epithelial damage. If a defective innate immune response plays a role in this disease (as in the hypothesis described above), it is possible that failure to clear bacteria from sites of injury allow increased permeability to occur, which then predisposes to immune activation leading to infection.

The finding of increased permeability in healthy relatives has led researchers to suggest that the hyperpermeability may be a genetically driven primary defect.[198, 199] A recent study attempted to assess the genetic aspect of permeability in these patients[199]; increased permeability was found in Crohn's disease patients, as expected, but not in unrelated household members or controls. A high prevalence of NOD2 (CARD15) mutations was found in patients and relatives compared to controls. And in the healthy relatives, high permeability and the presence of a NOD2 polymorphism were significantly associated.[199]

Immune dysregulation — There is also evidence to suggest that Crohn's disease is characterized by a loss of tolerance that leads to an excessive Th1 cell response to normal enteric bacteria.[6] Lack of appropriate numbers of regulatory T cells due to lack of stimulation by helminths (which are no longer present in our flora) has also been suggested to play a part.[275] Other organisms that serve as adjuvants for regulatory T cell induction include saprophytic *Mycobacterium* and *Lactobacillus* species.

Type 1 Diabetes

There is increasing evidence that alterations in gut flora and permeability are associated with type 1 diabetes. It has long been known that type 1 diabetes results from an interaction between genetic and environmental factors, but the rising incidence over the last several decades has led at least some researchers to conclude that environmental factors are increasingly involved in the pathogenesis and may be more important than genetic predisposition.[276]

Dysbiosis — Recent studies have attempted to assess the role of gut flora in the pathogenesis of diabetes. Analysis of gut flora of Bio-Breeding diabetes-prone rats showed that rats developing diabetes had increased levels of *Bifidobacterium* species in the gut.[277] Furthermore, in another experiment with Bio-Breeding diabetes-prone rats, antibiotic treatment decreased the total gut bacterial count and both delayed the subsequent development of diabetes and decreased the number of rats developing disease. Combining antibiotic treatment with a diet high in hydrolyzed casein completely protected against the development of diabetes.[277] This effect of antibiotics was also observed in another study on the non-obese diabetic mouse.[235] Furthermore, administration of oral probiotics has been shown to prevent the development of diabetes in mice.[278] (A large trial is under way to examine whether the administration of probiotics during the first 6 months of life will decrease the incidence of diabetes in high-risk populations.[279]) And in another study, gastrointestinal inoculation with helminths (*Trichinella spiralis* or *Heligmosomoides polygyrus*) inhibited the development of diabetes in mice.[280]

Permeability — Increases in gut permeability may also play a role in the development of type 1 diabetes, possibly in conjunction with alterations in gut flora. In a recent study, upregulation of zonulin, one of the proteins involved in modulating tight junction integrity, was associated with increases in permeability both in patients with type 1 diabetes and in their healthy relatives.[281] In another study, increases in permeability were found to precede the onset of diabetes.[234] It is not yet clear whether the vulnerability to increased permeability is inherited (as it may be in Crohn's disease) or whether it is the result of some other factor.

Immune dysregulation — Together, this evidence suggests that alterations in gut flora and/or permeability are allowing access of certain antigens to the GALT and thereby initiating autoimmunity. A recent report hypothesized that dietary bovine insulin, a "modified self-antigen" differing by only 3 amino acids from human insulin and present in cow's milk, acts as the trigger for the production of antibodies against both the bovine insulin and the host insulin-producing β-cells.[282] That author's hypothesis is that gut inflammation, caused by enteral infections or possibly gluten, activates immunity to dietary insulin and pancreatic cells, whereas other factors support the development of tolerance to insulin, such as breast-feeding and the development of healthy gut flora.[282]

Indeed, there seems to be an association between early exposure to cow's milk, short duration of breast-feeding, and the development of diabetes.[283] Specific proliferation of T-lymphocytes with bovine β-casein has been found in patients with recent-onset type 1 diabetes; this finding, in association with the known homology between bovine β-casein and molecules expressed on pancreatic β-cells, leads the authors to suggest that exposure to cow's milk may trigger a cellular and humoral response to bovine β-casein and also to self-antigens expressed on pancreatic β-cells.[284] A large study is under way to assess the effect of weaning to hydrolyzed casein rather than to conventional cow's milk on the subsequent development of diabetes.[285]

The association of type 1 diabetes with celiac disease (discussed in Chapter 1) provides further evidence that gut permeability defects (either primary or secondary) and immune responses to dietary antigens may be central to the development of both diseases.

Summary

The gastrointestinal immune system is critical to maintaining human health. It involves complex interactions between gut flora, gut epithelial cell junctions, and immune cells. Disruptions to this complex system are common in modern life, induced by factors such as diet, drugs, stress, and infection. Genetic predisposition also plays a role in the pathogenesis of diseases associated with changes in gut flora and gut permeability. Disturbances in the complex interactions between gut flora, permeability, and the GALT have great clinical relevance, as they have been implicated in the pathogenesis of, or susceptibility to, many serious chronic diseases, including numerous atopic and autoimmune diseases and their complications.

References

1. Bengmark S. Prospects for new and rediscovered therapies: probiotics and phage. In: Andrew PW, Oyston P, Smith GL, Stewart-Tull DE, eds. *Fighting Infection in the 21st Century*. Malden, MA: Blackwell Science Ltd.; 2000:97-132.
2. Podolsky S. Cultural divergence: Elie Metchnikoff's Bacillus bulgaricus therapy and his underlying concept of health. *Bull Hist Med.* 1998;72:1-27.
3. Guarner F. Enteric flora in health and disease. *Digestion.* 2006;73 Suppl 1:5-12.
4. Ramakrishna BS. The normal bacterial flora of the human intestine and its regulation. *J Clin Gastroenterol.* 2007;41 Suppl 1:S2-6.
5. Macpherson AJ, Harris NL. Interactions between commensal intestinal bacteria and the immune system. *Nat Rev Immunol.* 2004;4:478-485.
6. Balfour Sartor R. Bacteria in Crohn's disease: mechanisms of inflammation and therapeutic implications. *J Clin Gastroenterol.* 2007;41 Suppl 1: S37-43.
7. Mueller C, Macpherson AJ. Layers of mutualism with commensal bacteria protect us from intestinal inflammation. *Gut.* 2006;55:276-284.
8. Lukaczer D, Jones DS, Lerman RH. Digestion, absorption, and gut ecology. *Clinical Nutrition: A Functional Approach.* Gig Harbor, WA: The Institute for Functional Medicine; 2004:191-214.
9. Winkler P, Ghadimi D, Schrezenmeir J, Kraehenbuhl JP. Molecular and cellular basis of microflora-host interactions. *J Nutr.* 2007;137:756S-772S.
10. Taupin D, Podolsky DK. Trefoil factors: initiators of mucosal healing. *Nat Rev Mol Cell Biol.* 2003;4:721-732.
11. Corthesy B. Roundtrip ticket for secretory IgA: role in mucosal homeostasis? *J Immunol.* 2007;178:27-32.
12. Fasano A. Regulation of intercellular tight junctions by zonula occludens toxin and its eukaryotic analogue zonulin. *Ann N Y Acad Sci.* 2000;915:214-222.
13. Mowat AM. Anatomical basis of tolerance and immunity to intestinal antigens. *Nat Rev Immunol.* 2003;3:331-341.

14. Dahan S, Roth-Walter F, Arnaboldi P, Agarwal S, Mayer L. Epithelia: lymphocyte interactions in the gut. *Immunol Rev.* 2007;215:243-253.
15. Iweala OI, Nagler CR. Immune privilege in the gut: the establishment and maintenance of non-responsiveness to dietary antigens and commensal flora. *Immunol Rev.* 2006;213:82-100.
16. O'Hara AM, Shanahan F. The gut flora as a forgotten organ. *EMBO Rep.* 2006;7:688-693.
17. Barbara G, Stanghellini V, Brandi G, et al. Interactions between commensal bacteria and gut sensorimotor function in health and disease. *Am J Gastroenterol.* 2005;100:2560-2568.
18. Clayburgh DR, Shen L, Turner JR. A porous defense: the leaky epithelial barrier in intestinal disease. *Lab Invest.* 2004;84:282-291.
19. Baumgart DC, Dignass AU. Intestinal barrier function. *Curr Opin Clin Nutr Metab Care.* 2002;5:685-694.
20. Menconi MJ, Salzman AL, Unno N, et al. Acidosis induces hyperpermeability in Caco-2BBe cultured intestinal epithelial monolayers. *Am J Physiol.* 1997;272:G1007-1021.
21. Maher S, Feighery L, Brayden DJ, McClean S. Melittin as an epithelial permeability enhancer I: investigation of its mechanism of action in caco-2 monolayers. *Pharm Res.* 2007;24:1336-1345.
22. Ohata A, Usami M, Miyoshi M. Short-chain fatty acids alter tight junction permeability in intestinal monolayer cells via lipoxygenase activation. *Nutrition.* 2005;21:838-847.
23. Blikslager AT, Roberts MC, Rhoads JM, Argenzio RA. Prostaglandins I2 and E2 have a synergistic role in rescuing epithelial barrier function in porcine ileum. *J Clin Invest.* 1997;100:1928-1933.
24. Blikslager AT, Moeser AJ, Gookin JL, Jones SL, Odle J. Restoration of barrier function in injured intestinal mucosa. *Physiol Rev.* 2007;87:545-564.
25. Savidge TC, Newman P, Pothoulakis C, et al. Enteric glia regulate intestinal barrier function and inflammation via release of S-nitrosoglutathione. *Gastroenterology.* 2007;132:1344-1358.
26. Madara J. Building an intestine--architectural contributions of commensal bacteria. *N Engl J Med.* 2004;351:1685-1686.
27. Kidd P. Th1/Th2 balance: the hypothesis, its limitations, and implications for health and disease. *Altern Med Rev.* 2003;8:223-246.
28. Weiner HL. Oral tolerance: immune mechanisms and the generation of Th3-type TGF-beta-secreting regulatory cells. *Microbes Infect.* 2001;3:947-954.
29. Chen Z, O'Shea JJ. Th17 cells: a new fate for differentiating helper T cells. *Immunol Res.* 2008.
30. Gardner ML. Gastrointestinal absorption of intact proteins. *Annu Rev Nutr.* 1988;8:329-350.
31. Macdonald TT, Monteleone G. Immunity, inflammation, and allergy in the gut. *Science.* 2005;307:1920-1925.
32. Steinhoff U. Who controls the crowd? New findings and old questions about the intestinal microflora. *Immunol Lett.* 2005;99:12-16.
33. Van Parijs L, Abbas AK. Homeostasis and self-tolerance in the immune system: turning lymphocytes off. *Science.* 1998;280:243-248.
34. Kronmal RA, McClelland RL, Detrano R, et al. Risk factors for the progression of coronary artery calcification in asymptomatic subjects: results from the Multi-Ethnic Study of Atherosclerosis (MESA). *Circulation.* 2007;115:2722-2730.
35. Enzinger PC, Mayer RJ. Esophageal cancer. *N Engl J Med.* 2003;349:2241-2252.
36. McGarr SE, Ridlon JM, Hylemon PB. Diet, anaerobic bacterial metabolism, and colon cancer: a review of the literature. *J Clin Gastroenterol.* 2005;39:98-109.
37. Kay AB. Allergy and allergic diseases. First of two parts. *N Engl J Med.* 2001;344:30-37.
38. Hanauer SB. Inflammatory bowel disease: epidemiology, pathogenesis, and therapeutic opportunities. *Inflamm Bowel Dis.* 2006;12 Suppl 1:S3-9.
39. Cooper GS, Stroehla BC. The epidemiology of autoimmune diseases. *Autoimmun Rev.* 2003;2:119-125.
40. Reiss AB, Glass AD. Atherosclerosis: immune and inflammatory aspects. *J Investig Med.* 2006;54:123-131.
41. Fox JG, Wang TC. Inflammation, atrophy, and gastric cancer. *J Clin Invest.* 2007;117:60-69.
42. Lagergren J, Bergstrom R, Lindgren A, Nyren O. Symptomatic gastroesophageal reflux as a risk factor for esophageal adenocarcinoma. *N Engl J Med.* 1999;340:825-831.
43. Itzkowitz SH, Yio X. Inflammation and cancer IV. Colorectal cancer in inflammatory bowel disease: the role of inflammation. *Am J Physiol Gastrointest Liver Physiol.* 2004;287:G7-17.
44. O'Byrne KJ, Dalgleish AG. Chronic immune activation and inflammation as the cause of malignancy. *Br J Cancer.* 2001;85:473-483.
45. Murray M, Pizzorno J. *Encyclopedia of Natural Medicine.* Rocklin, CA: Prima Publishing; 1998.
46. Fujinami RS, von Herrath MG, Christen U, Whitton JL. Molecular mimicry, bystander activation, or viral persistence: infections and autoimmune disease. *Clin Microbiol Rev.* 2006;19:80-94.
47. Fasano A, Shea-Donohue T. Mechanisms of disease: the role of intestinal barrier function in the pathogenesis of gastrointestinal autoimmune diseases. *Nat Clin Pract Gastroenterol Hepatol.* 2005;2:416-422.
48. Guarner F, Bourdet-Sicard R, Brandtzaeg P, et al. Mechanisms of disease: the hygiene hypothesis revisited. *Nat Clin Pract Gastroenterol Hepatol.* 2006;3:275-284.
49. Hebuterne X. Gut changes attributed to ageing: effects on intestinal microflora. *Curr Opin Clin Nutr Metab Care.* 2003;6:49-54.
50. Hopkins MJ, Sharp R, Macfarlane GT. Variation in human intestinal microbiota with age. *Dig Liver Dis.* 2002;34 Suppl 2:S12-18.
51. Westerbeek EA, van den Berg A, Lafeber HN, Knol J, Fetter WP, van Elburg RM. The intestinal bacterial colonisation in preterm infants: a review of the literature. *Clin Nutr.* 2006;25:361-368.
52. Woodmansey EJ. Intestinal bacteria and ageing. *J Appl Microbiol.* 2007;102:1178-1186.
53. Hopkins MJ, Sharp R, Macfarlane GT. Age and disease related changes in intestinal bacterial populations assessed by cell culture, 16S rRNA abundance, and community cellular fatty acid profiles. *Gut.* 2001;48:198-205.
54. Hopkins MJ, Macfarlane GT. Changes in predominant bacterial populations in human faeces with age and with Clostridium difficile infection. *J Med Microbiol.* 2002;51:448-454.
55. Holt PR. Intestinal malabsorption in the elderly. *Dig Dis.* 2007;25:144-150.
56. Chang C, Miller JF. Campylobacter jejuni colonization of mice with limited enteric flora. *Infect Immun.* 2006;74:5261-5271.
57. Almeida J, Galhenage S, Yu J, Kurtovic J, Riordan SM. Gut flora and bacterial translocation in chronic liver disease. *World J Gastroenterol.* 2006;12:1493-1502.
58. Bhattacharya A, Anand MT, Paul J, Yadav N, Bhattacharya S. Molecular changes in Entamoeba histolytica in response to bacteria. *J Eukaryot Microbiol.* 1998;45:28S-33S.
59. Reid G, Burton J. Use of Lactobacillus to prevent infection by pathogenic bacteria. *Microbes Infect.* 2002;4:319-324.
60. Ivec M, Botic T, Koren S, Jakobsen M, Weingartl H, Cencic A. Interactions of macrophages with probiotic bacteria lead to increased antiviral response against vesicular stomatitis virus. *Antiviral Res.* 2007;75:266-274.

61. Hammerman C, Kaplan M. Probiotics and neonatal intestinal infection. *Curr Opin Infect Dis.* 2006;19:277-282.
62. McFarland LV. Meta-analysis of probiotics for the prevention of antibiotic associated diarrhea and the treatment of Clostridium difficile disease. *Am J Gastroenterol.* 2006;101:812-822.
63. Besselink MG, van Santvoort HC, Buskens E, et al. Probiotic prophylaxis in predicted severe acute pancreatitis: a randomised, double-blind, placebo-controlled trial. *Lancet.* 2008;371:651-659.
64. Rani R, Murthy RS, Bhattacharya S, Ahuja V, Rizvi MA, Paul J. Changes in bacterial profile during amebiasis: demonstration of anaerobic bacteria in ALA pus samples. *Am J Trop Med Hyg.* 2006;75:880-885.
65. Cummings JH, Macfarlane GT. Role of intestinal bacteria in nutrient metabolism. *JPEN J Parenter Enteral Nutr.* 1997;21:357-365.
66. Clavel T, Fallani M, Lepage P, et al. Isoflavones and functional foods alter the dominant intestinal microbiota in postmenopausal women. *J Nutr.* 2005;135:2786-2792.
67. Gueimonde M, Laitinen K, Salminen S, Isolauri E. Breast milk: a source of bifidobacteria for infant gut development and maturation? *Neonatology.* 2007;92:64-66.
68. Fanaro S, Chierici R, Guerrini P, Vigi V. Intestinal microflora in early infancy: composition and development. *Acta Paediatr Suppl.* 2003;91:48-55.
69. Edwards CA, Parrett AM. Intestinal flora during the first months of life: new perspectives. *Br J Nutr.* 2002;88 Suppl 1:S11-18.
70. Gibson GR, Roberfroid MB. Dietary modulation of the human colonic microbiota: introducing the concept of prebiotics. *J Nutr.* 1995;125:1401-1412.
71. Roy CC, Kien CL, Bouthillier L, Levy E. Short-chain fatty acids: ready for prime time? *Nutr Clin Pract.* 2006;21:351-366.
72. Gibson GR, Beatty ER, Wang X, Cummings JH. Selective stimulation of bifidobacteria in the human colon by oligofructose and inulin. *Gastroenterology.* 1995;108:975 982.
73. Gostner A, Blaut M, Schaffer V, et al. Effect of isomalt consumption on faecal microflora and colonic metabolism in healthy volunteers. *Br J Nutr.* 2006;95:40-50.
74. Ohkusa T, Ozaki Y, Sato C, Mikuni K, Ikeda H. Long-term ingestion of lactosucrose increases Bifidobacterium sp. in human fecal flora. *Digestion.* 1995;56:415-420.
75. Bouhnik Y, Raskine L, Simoneau G, et al. The capacity of nondigestible carbohydrates to stimulate fecal bifidobacteria in healthy humans: a double-blind, randomized, placebo-controlled, parallel-group, dose-response relation study. *Am J Clin Nutr.* 2004;80:1658-1664.
76. Kleessen B, Sykura B, Zunft HJ, Blaut M. Effects of inulin and lactose on fecal microflora, microbial activity, and bowel habit in elderly constipated persons. *Am J Clin Nutr.* 1997;65:1397-1402.
77. Zentek J, Marquart B, Pietrzak T, Ballevre O, Rochat F. Dietary effects on bifidobacteria and Clostridium perfringens in the canine intestinal tract. *J Anim Physiol Anim Nutr (Berl).* 2003;87:397-407.
78. Apajalahti JH, Kettunen H, Kettunen A, et al. Culture-independent microbial community analysis reveals that inulin in the diet primarily affects previously unknown bacteria in the mouse cecum. *Appl Environ Microbiol.* 2002;68:4986-4995.
79. Kleessen B, Stoof G, Proll J, Schmiedl D, Noack J, Blaut M. Feeding resistant starch affects fecal and cecal microflora and short-chain fatty acids in rats. *J Anim Sci.* 1997;75:2453-2462.
80. Silvi S, Rumney CJ, Cresci A, Rowland IR. Resistant starch modifies gut microflora and microbial metabolism in human flora-associated rats inoculated with faeces from Italian and UK donors. *J Appl Microbiol.* 1999;86:521-530.
81. Loh G, Eberhard M, Brunner RM, et al. Inulin alters the intestinal microbiota and short-chain fatty acid concentrations in growing pigs regardless of their basal diet. *J Nutr.* 2006;136:1198-1202.
82. Kleessen B, Blaut M. Modulation of gut mucosal biofilms. *Br J Nutr.* 2005;93 Suppl 1:S35-40.
83. Bjerrum L, Pedersen AB, Engberg RM. The influence of whole wheat feeding on Salmonella infection and gut flora composition in broilers. *Avian Dis.* 2005;49:9-15.
84. van Faassen A, Bol J, van Dokkum W, Pikaar NA, Ockhuizen T, Hermus RJ. Bile acids, neutral steroids, and bacteria in feces as affected by a mixed, a lacto-ovovegetarian, and a vegan diet. *Am J Clin Nutr.* 1987;46:962-967.
85. Peltonen R, Ling WH, Hanninen O, Eerola E. An uncooked vegan diet shifts the profile of human fecal microflora: computerized analysis of direct stool sample gas-liquid chromatography profiles of bacterial cellular fatty acids. *Appl Environ Microbiol.* 1992;58:3660-3666.
86. Noack-Loebel C, Kuster E, Rusch V, Zimmermann K. Influence of different dietary regimens upon the composition of the human fecal flora. *Prog Food Nutr Sci.* 1983;7:127-131.
87. Christl SU, Gibson GR, Cummings JH. Role of dietary sulphate in the regulation of methanogenesis in the human large intestine. *Gut.* 1992;33:1234-1238.
88. Wells JE, Berr F, Thomas LA, Dowling RH, Hylemon PB. Isolation and characterization of cholic acid 7alpha-dehydroxylating fecal bacteria from cholesterol gallstone patients. *J Hepatol.* 2000;32:4-10.
89. Uchida K, Satoh T, Narushima S, et al. Transformation of bile acids and sterols by clostridia (fusiform bacteria) in Wistar rats. *Lipids.* 1999;34:269-273.
90. Watabe J, Bernstein H. The mutagenicity of bile acids using a fluctuation test. *Mutat Res.* 1985;158:45-51.
91. O'Keefe SJ, Chung D, Mahmoud N, et al. Why do African Americans get more colon cancer than Native Africans? *J Nutr.* 2007;137:175S-182S.
92. Mensah PP, Tomkins AM, Drasar BS, Harrison TJ. Effect of fermentation of Ghanaian maize dough on the survival and proliferation of 4 strains of Shigella flexneri. *Trans R Soc Trop Med Hyg.* 1988;82:635-636.
93. Akil I, Yilmaz O, Kurutepe S, Degerli K, Kavukcu S. Influence of oral intake of Saccharomyces boulardii on Escherichia coli in enteric flora. *Pediatr Nephrol.* 2006;21:807-810.
94. Haskel Y, Udassin R, Freund HR, Zhang JM, Hanani M. Liquid enteral diets induce bacterial translocation by increasing cecal flora without changing intestinal motility. *JPEN J Parenter Enteral Nutr.* 2001;25:60-64.
95. Schneider SM, Le Gall P, Girard-Pipau F, et al. Total artificial nutrition is associated with major changes in the fecal flora. *Eur J Nutr.* 2000;39:248-255.
96. Gismondo MR. Antibiotic impact on intestinal microflora. *Gastroenterol Int.* 1998;11:29-30.
97. Hentges DJ. Role of the intestinal microflora in host defense against infection. In: Hentges DJ, ed. *Human Intestinal Microflora in Health and Disease.* New York, NY: Academic Press; 1983:311-331.
98. Treinen-Moslen M, Kanz MF. Intestinal tract injury by drugs: Importance of metabolite delivery by yellow bile road. *Pharmacol Ther.* 2006;112:649-667.
99. Nord CE. Studies on the ecological impact of antibiotics. *Eur J Clin Microbiol Infect Dis.* 1990;9:517-518.

100. Nord CE, Edlund C. Impact of antimicrobial agents on human intestinal microflora. *J Chemother.* 1990;2:218-237.
101. Karachalios G, Charalabopoulos K. Biliary excretion of antimicrobial drugs. *Chemotherapy.* 2002;48:280-297.
102. Kilkkinen A, Pietinen P, Klaukka T, Virtamo J, Korhonen P, Adlercreutz H. Use of oral antimicrobials decreases serum enterolactone concentration. *Am J Epidemiol.* 2002;155:472-477.
103. Hawrelak JA, Myers SP. The causes of intestinal dysbiosis: a review. *Altern Med Rev.* 2004;9:180-197.
104. Bashford JN, Norwood J, Chapman SR. Why are patients prescribed proton pump inhibitors? Retrospective analysis of link between morbidity and prescribing in the General Practice Research Database. *Bmj.* 1998;317:452-456.
105. Williams C, McColl KE. Review article: proton pump inhibitors and bacterial overgrowth. *Aliment Pharmacol Ther.* 2006;23:3-10.
106. Nieuwenhuijs VB, Verheem A, van Duijvenbode-Beumer H, et al. The role of interdigestive small bowel motility in the regulation of gut microflora, bacterial overgrowth, and bacterial translocation in rats. *Ann Surg.* 1998;228:188-193.
107. Cappell MS. Colonic toxicity of administered drugs and chemicals. *Am J Gastroenterol.* 2004;99:1175-1190.
108. Panganamamula KV, Parkman HP. Chronic Intestinal Pseudo-Obstruction. *Curr Treat Options Gastroenterol.* 2005;8:3-11.
109. Catnach SM, Fairclough PD. Erythromycin and the gut. *Gut.* 1992;33:397-401.
110. Bode C, Bode JC. Effect of alcohol consumption on the gut. *Best Pract Res Clin Gastroenterol.* 2003;17:575-592.
111. Khalif IL, Quigley EM, Konovitch EA, Maximova ID. Alterations in the colonic flora and intestinal permeability and evidence of immune activation in chronic constipation. *Dig Liver Dis.* 2005;37:838-849.
112. Hart A, Kamm MA. Review article: mechanisms of initiation and perpetuation of gut inflammation by stress. *Aliment Pharmacol Ther.* 2002;16:2017-2028.
113. Bailey MT, Coe CL. Maternal separation disrupts the integrity of the intestinal microflora in infant rhesus monkeys. *Dev Psychobiol.* 1999;35:146-155.
114. Spitz JC, Ghandi S, Taveras M, Aoys E, Alverdy JC. Characteristics of the intestinal epithelial barrier during dietary manipulation and glucocorticoid stress. *Crit Care Med.* 1996;24:635-641.
115. Velin AK, Ericson AC, Braaf Y, Wallon C, Soderholm JD. Increased antigen and bacterial uptake in follicle associated epithelium induced by chronic psychological stress in rats. *Gut.* 2004;53:494-500.
116. Freestone PP, Williams PH, Haigh RD, Maggs AF, Neal CP, Lyte M. Growth stimulation of intestinal commensal Escherichia coli by catecholamines: a possible contributory factor in trauma-induced sepsis. *Shock.* 2002;18:465-470.
117. Freestone PP, Haigh RD, Lyte M. Specificity of catecholamine-induced growth in Escherichia coli O157:H7, Salmonella enterica and Yersinia enterocolitica. *FEMS Microbiol Lett.* 2007;269:221-228.
118. Holdeman LV, Good IJ, Moore WE. Human fecal flora: variation in bacterial composition within individuals and a possible effect of emotional stress. *Appl Environ Microbiol.* 1976;31:359-375.
119. Lizko NN. Stress and intestinal microflora. *Nahrung.* 1987;31:443-447.
120. Fedwick JP, Lapointe TK, Meddings JB, Sherman PM, Buret AG. Helicobacter pylori activates myosin light-chain kinase to disrupt claudin-4 and claudin-5 and increase epithelial permeability. *Infect Immun.* 2005;73:7844-7852.
121. Frank CF, Hostetter MK. Cleavage of E-cadherin: a mechanism for disruption of the intestinal epithelial barrier by Candida albicans. *Transl Res.* 2007;149:211-222.
122. Nyakundi JN, Crawley B, Pentreath VW. The relationships between endotoxins, nitric oxide and inflammatory cytokines in blood and intestinal tissues in experimental Trypanosoma brucei brucei infections. *Parasitology.* 2002;124:597-604.
123. Rollins NC, Filteau SM, Coutsoudis A, Tomkins AM. Feeding mode, intestinal permeability, and neopterin excretion: a longitudinal study in infants of HIV-infected South African women. *J Acquir Immune Defic Syndr.* 2001;28:132-139.
124. Tafazoli F, Holmstrom A, Forsberg A, Magnusson KE. Apically exposed, tight junction-associated beta1-integrins allow binding and YopE-mediated perturbation of epithelial barriers by wild-type Yersinia bacteria. *Infect Immun.* 2000;68:5335-5343.
125. Zhang Y, Lee B, Thompson M, et al. Lactulose-mannitol intestinal permeability test in children with diarrhea caused by rotavirus and cryptosporidium. Diarrhea Working Group, Peru. *J Pediatr Gastroenterol Nutr.* 2000;31:16-21.
126. Heyman M. Gut barrier dysfunction in food allergy. *Eur J Gastroenterol Hepatol.* 2005;17:1279-1285.
127. Hayashi M, Tomita M. Mechanistic analysis for drug permeation through intestinal membrane. *Drug Metab Pharmacokinet.* 2007;22:67-77.
128. Nchito M, Friis H, Michaelsen KF, Mubila L, Olsen A. Iron supplementation increases small intestine permeability in primary schoolchildren in Lusaka, Zambia. *Trans R Soc Trop Med Hyg.* 2006;100:791-794.
129. Parfitt JR, Driman DK. Pathological effects of drugs on the gastrointestinal tract: a review. *Hum Pathol.* 2007;38:527-536.
130. Barclay GR, Turnberg LA. Effect of cold-induced pain on salt and water transport in the human jejunum. *Gastroenterology.* 1988;94:994-998.
131. Santos J, Saperas E, Nogueiras C, et al. Release of mast cell mediators into the jejunum by cold pain stress in humans. *Gastroenterology.* 1998;114:640-648.
132. Indrio F, Raimondi F, Laforgia N, Riezzo G, Polimeno L, Francavilla R. Effect of hyperbilirubinemia on intestinal permeability in healthy term newborns. *Acta Paediatr.* 2007;96:73-75.
133. Raimondi F, Crivaro V, Capasso L, et al. Unconjugated bilirubin modulates the intestinal epithelial barrier function in a human-derived in vitro model. *Pediatr Res.* 2006;60:30-33.
134. Assimakopoulos SF, Vagianos CE, Charonis AS, et al. Experimental obstructive jaundice alters claudin-4 expression in intestinal mucosa: effect of bombesin and neurotensin. *World J Gastroenterol.* 2006;12:3410-3415.
135. Buchman AL, Moukarzel AA, Bhuta S, et al. Parenteral nutrition is associated with intestinal morphologic and functional changes in humans. *JPEN J Parenter Enteral Nutr.* 1995;19:453-460.
136. van Elburg RM, Fetter WP, Bunkers CM, Heymans HS. Intestinal permeability in relation to birth weight and gestational and postnatal age. *Arch Dis Child Fetal Neonatal Ed.* 2003;88:F52-55.
137. Rouwet EV, Heineman E, Buurman WA, ter Riet G, Ramsay G, Blanco CE. Intestinal permeability and carrier-mediated monosaccharide absorption in preterm neonates during the early postnatal period. *Pediatr Res.* 2002;51:64-70.
138. Mullin JM, Valenzano MC, Verrecchio JJ, Kothari R. Age- and diet-related increase in transepithelial colon permeability of Fischer 344 rats. *Dig Dis Sci.* 2002;47:2262-2270.
139. Saltzman JR, Kowdley KV, Perrone G, Russell RM. Changes in small-intestine permeability with aging. *J Am Geriatr Soc.* 1995;43:160-164.
140. Montalto M, Maggiano N, Ricci R, et al. Lactobacillus acidophilus protects tight junctions from aspirin damage in HT-29 cells. *Digestion.* 2004;69:225-228.

141. Ait-Belgnaoui A, Han W, Lamine F, et al. Lactobacillus farciminis treatment suppresses stress induced visceral hypersensitivity: a possible action through interaction with epithelial cell cytoskeleton contraction. *Gut.* 2006;55:1090-1094.
142. Zyrek AA, Cichon C, Helms S, Enders C, Sonnenborn U, Schmidt MA. Molecular mechanisms underlying the probiotic effects of Escherichia coli Nissle 1917 involve ZO-2 and PKCzeta redistribution resulting in tight junction and epithelial barrier repair. *Cell Microbiol.* 2007;9:804-816.
143. Commane DM, Shortt CT, Silvi S, Cresci A, Hughes RM, Rowland IR. Effects of fermentation products of pro- and prebiotics on trans-epithelial electrical resistance in an in vitro model of the colon. *Nutr Cancer.* 2005;51:102-109.
144. Bai YH, Pak SC, Lee SH, et al. Assessment of a bioactive compound for its potential antiinflammatory property by tight junction permeability. *Phytother Res.* 2005;19:1009-1012.
145. Garcia-Lafuente A, Antolin M, Guarner F, Crespo E, Malagelada JR. Modulation of colonic barrier function by the composition of the commensal flora in the rat. *Gut.* 2001;48:503-507.
146. Heyman M, Terpend K, Menard S. Effects of specific lactic acid bacteria on the intestinal permeability to macromolecules and the inflammatory condition. *Acta Paediatr Suppl.* 2005;94:34-36.
147. Mariadason JM, Barkla DH, Gibson PR. Effect of short-chain fatty acids on paracellular permeability in Caco-2 intestinal epithelium model. *Am J Physiol.* 1997;272:G705-712.
148. Ventura MT, Polimeno L, Amoruso AC, et al. Intestinal permeability in patients with adverse reactions to food. *Dig Liver Dis.* 2006;38:732-736.
149. Colome G, Sierra C, Blasco J, Garcia MV, Valverde E, Sanchez E. Intestinal permeability in different feedings in infancy. *Acta Paediatr.* 2007;96:69-72.
150. Duffy LC. Interactions mediating bacterial translocation in the immature intestine. *J Nutr.* 2000;130:432S-436S.
151. Townsend S, Caubilla Barron J, Loc-Carrillo C, Forsythe S. The presence of endotoxin in powdered infant formula milk and the influence of endotoxin and Enterobacter sakazakii on bacterial translocation in the infant rat. *Food Microbiol.* 2007;24:67-74.
152. Bjorkman DJ. Nonsteroidal anti-inflammatory drug-induced gastrointestinal injury. *Am J Med.* 1996;101:25S-32S.
153. Singh G. Gastrointestinal complications of prescription and over-the-counter nonsteroidal anti-inflammatory drugs: a view from the ARAMIS database. Arthritis, Rheumatism, and Aging Medical Information System. *Am J Ther.* 2000;7:115-121.
154. Lanas A, Scarpignato C. Microbial flora in NSAID-induced intestinal damage: a role for antibiotics? *Digestion.* 2006;73 Suppl 1:136-150.
155. Fortun PJ, Hawkey CJ. Nonsteroidal antiinflammatory drugs and the small intestine. *Curr Opin Gastroenterol.* 2007;23:134-141.
156. Maiden L, Thjodleifsson B, Theodors A, Gonzalez J, Bjarnason I. A quantitative analysis of NSAID-induced small bowel pathology by capsule enteroscopy. *Gastroenterology.* 2005;128:1172-1178.
157. Graham DY, Opekun AR, Willingham FF, Qureshi WA. Visible small-intestinal mucosal injury in chronic NSAID users. *Clin Gastroenterol Hepatol.* 2005;3:55-59.
158. Laine L, Smith R, Min K, Chen C, Dubois RW. Systematic review: the lower gastrointestinal adverse effects of non-steroidal anti-inflammatory drugs. *Aliment Pharmacol Ther.* 2006;24:751-767.
159. Byrne MF, McGuinness J, Smyth CM, et al. Nonsteroidal anti-inflammatory drug-induced diaphragms and ulceration in the colon. *Eur J Gastroenterol Hepatol.* 2002;14:1265-1269.
160. Thiefin G, Beaugerie L. Toxic effects of nonsteroidal antiinflammatory drugs on the small bowel, colon, and rectum. *Joint Bone Spine.* 2005;72:286-294.
161. Laine L, Connors LG, Reicin A, et al. Serious lower gastrointestinal clinical events with nonselective NSAID or coxib use. *Gastroenterology.* 2003;124:288-292.
162. Sigthorsson G, Simpson RJ, Walley M, et al. COX-1 and 2, intestinal integrity, and pathogenesis of nonsteroidal anti-inflammatory drug enteropathy in mice. *Gastroenterology.* 2002;122:1913-1923.
163. Leung WK, Bjarnason I, Wong VW, Sung JJ, Chan FK. Small bowel enteropathy associated with chronic low-dose aspirin therapy. *Lancet.* 2007;369:614.
164. Manetas M, O'Loughlin C, Kelemen K, Barkin JS. Multiple small-bowel diaphragms: a cause of obscure GI bleeding diagnosed by capsule endoscopy. *Gastrointest Endosc.* 2004;60:848-851.
165. Montalto M, Curigliano V, Santoro L, et al. Prophylactic aspirin therapy does not increase faecal calprotectin concentrations. *Eur J Gastroenterol Hepatol.* 2006;18:965-967.
166. Campbell CL, Smyth S, Montalescot G, Steinhubl SR. Aspirin dose for the prevention of cardiovascular disease: a systematic review. *Jama.* 2007;297:2018-2024.
167. Ajani UA, Ford ES, Greenland KJ, Giles WH, Mokdad AH. Aspirin use among U.S. adults: Behavioral Risk Factor Surveillance System. *Am J Prev Med.* 2006;30:74-77.
168. Hond ED, Peeters M, Hiele M, Bulteel V, Ghoos Y, Rutgeerts P. Effect of glutamine on the intestinal permeability changes induced by indomethacin in humans. *Aliment Pharmacol Ther.* 1999;13:679-685.
169. Playford RJ, MacDonald CE, Calnan DP, et al. Co-administration of the health food supplement, bovine colostrum, reduces the acute non-steroidal anti-inflammatory drug-induced increase in intestinal permeability. *Clin Sci (Lond).* 2001;100:627-633.
170. Yang PC, Jury J, Soderholm JD, Sherman PM, McKay DM, Perdue MH. Chronic psychological stress in rats induces intestinal sensitization to luminal antigens. *Am J Pathol.* 2006;168:104-114; quiz 363.
171. Soderholm JD, Yang PC, Ceponis P, et al. Chronic stress induces mast cell-dependent bacterial adherence and initiates mucosal inflammation in rat intestine. *Gastroenterology.* 2002;123:1099-1108.
172. Saunders PR, Santos J, Hanssen NP, Yates D, Groot JA, Perdue MH. Physical and psychological stress in rats enhances colonic epithelial permeability via peripheral CRH. *Dig Dis Sci.* 2002;47:208-215.
173. Ponferrada A, Caso JR, Alou L, et al. The role of PPARgamma on restoration of colonic homeostasis after experimental stress-induced inflammation and dysfunction. *Gastroenterology.* 2007;132:1791-1803.
174. Bhatia V, Tandon RK. Stress and the gastrointestinal tract. *J Gastroenterol Hepatol.* 2005;20:332-339.
175. Barreau F, Cartier C, Leveque M, et al. Pathways involved in gut mucosal barrier dysfunction induced in adult rats by maternal deprivation: corticotrophin-releasing factor and nerve growth factor interplay. *J Physiol.* 2007;580:347-356.
176. Rashid T, Ebringer A. Ankylosing spondylitis is linked to Klebsiella-the evidence. *Clin Rheumatol.* 2007;26:858-864.
177. Rudwaleit M, Baeten D. Ankylosing spondylitis and bowel disease. *Best Pract Res Clin Rheumatol.* 2006;20:451-471.
178. Braun J, Sieper J. Ankylosing spondylitis. *Lancet.* 2007;369:1379-1390.
179. Reveille JD. Major histocompatibility genes and ankylosing spondylitis. *Best Pract Res Clin Rheumatol.* 2006;20:601-609.

180. Davies JM. Molecular mimicry: can epitope mimicry induce autoimmune disease? *Immunol Cell Biol.* 1997;75:113-126.
181. Schwimmbeck PL, Yu DT, Oldstone MB. Autoantibodies to HLA B27 in the sera of HLA B27 patients with ankylosing spondylitis and Reiter's syndrome. Molecular mimicry with Klebsiella pneumoniae as potential mechanism of autoimmune disease. *J Exp Med.* 1987;166:173-181.
182. Fielder M, Pirt SJ, Tarpey I, et al. Molecular mimicry and ankylosing spondylitis: possible role of a novel sequence in pullulanase of Klebsiella pneumoniae. *FEBS Lett.* 1995;369:243-248.
183. Charalambous BM, Keen JN, McPherson MJ. Collagen-like sequences stabilize homotrimers of a bacterial hydrolase. *Embo J.* 1988;7:2903-2909.
184. Wilson C, Rashid T, Tiwana H, et al. Cytotoxicity responses to peptide antigens in rheumatoid arthritis and ankylosing spondylitis. *J Rheumatol.* 2003;30:972-978.
185. Husby G, Tsuchiya N, Schwimmbeck PL, et al. Cross-reactive epitope with Klebsiella pneumoniae nitrogenase in articular tissue of HLA-B27+ patients with ankylosing spondylitis. *Arthritis Rheum.* 1989;32:437-445.
186. Martinez-Gonzalez O, Cantero-Hinojosa J, Paule-Sastre P, Gomez-Magan JC, Salvatierra-Rios D. Intestinal permeability in patients with ankylosing spondylitis and their healthy relatives. *Br J Rheumatol.* 1994;33:644-647.
187. Benitez-Del-Castillo JM, Garcia-Sanchez J, Iradier T, Banares A. Sulfasalazine in the prevention of anterior uveitis associated with ankylosing spondylitis. *Eye.* 2000;14 (Pt 3A):340-343.
188. Vaile JH, Meddings JB, Yacyshyn BR, Russell AS, Maksymowych WP. Bowel permeability and CD45RO expression on circulating CD20+ B cells in patients with ankylosing spondylitis and their relatives. *J Rheumatol.* 1999;26:128-135.
189. Kuiper S, van Pelt J, Verheesen PE, Rentsch HU, Stockbrugger R, van der Linden SM. Patients with ankylosing spondylitis and healthy relatives do not show increased small intestinal permeability with the lactulose-mannitol test. *Clin Exp Rheumatol.* 1993;11:413-416.
190. Ferraz MB, Atra E, Trabulsi LR, Goldenberg J, Sato EI. A study of the gram-negative bacterial flora in patients with ankylosing spondylitis. *Braz J Med Biol Res.* 1990;23:29-36.
191. Monsuur AJ, Wijmenga C. Understanding the molecular basis of celiac disease: what genetic studies reveal. *Ann Med.* 2006;38:578-591.
192. Nieuwenhuizen WF, Pieters RH, Knippels LM, Jansen MC, Koppelman SJ. Is Candida albicans a trigger in the onset of coeliac disease? *Lancet.* 2003;361:2152-2154.
193. Troncone R, Auricchio S. Rotavirus and celiac disease: clues to the pathogenesis and perspectives on prevention. *J Pediatr Gastroenterol Nutr.* 2007;44:527-528.
194. Forsberg G, Fahlgren A, Horstedt P, Hammarstrom S, Hernell O, Hammarstrom ML. Presence of bacteria and innate immunity of intestinal epithelium in childhood celiac disease. *Am J Gastroenterol.* 2004;99:894-904.
195. Rath HC, Schultz M, Freitag R, et al. Different subsets of enteric bacteria induce and perpetuate experimental colitis in rats and mice. *Infect Immun.* 2001;69:2277-2285.
196. Mylonaki M, Rayment NB, Rampton DS, Hudspith BN, Brostoff J. Molecular characterization of rectal mucosa-associated bacterial flora in inflammatory bowel disease. *Inflamm Bowel Dis.* 2005;11:481-487.
197. Ott SJ, Musfeldt M, Wenderoth DF, et al. Reduction in diversity of the colonic mucosa associated bacterial microflora in patients with active inflammatory bowel disease. *Gut.* 2004;53:685-693.
198. D'Inca R, Annese V, di Leo V, et al. Increased intestinal permeability and NOD2 variants in familial and sporadic Crohn's disease. *Aliment Pharmacol Ther.* 2006;23:1455-1461.
199. Buhner S, Buning C, Genschel J, et al. Genetic basis for increased intestinal permeability in families with Crohn's disease: role of CARD15 3020insC mutation? *Gut.* 2006;55:342-347.
200. Quaglietta L, te Velde A, Staiano A, Troncone R, Hommes DW. Functional consequences of NOD2/CARD15 mutations in Crohn disease. *J Pediatr Gastroenterol Nutr.* 2007;44:529-539.
201. Lala S, Ogura Y, Osborne C, et al. Crohn's disease and the NOD2 gene: a role for paneth cells. *Gastroenterology.* 2003;125:47-57.
202. Baumgart DC, Carding SR. Inflammatory bowel disease: cause and immunobiology. *Lancet.* 2007;369:1627-1640.
203. Podolsky DK. Inflammatory bowel disease. *N Engl J Med.* 2002;347:417-429.
204. Wills-Karp M, Ewart SL. Time to draw breath: asthma-susceptibility genes are identified. *Nat Rev Genet.* 2004;5:376-387.
205. Bowcock AM, Cookson WO. The genetics of psoriasis, psoriatic arthritis and atopic dermatitis. *Hum Mol Genet.* 2004;13 Spec No 1:R43-55.
206. Cookson W. The immunogenetics of asthma and eczema: a new focus on the epithelium. *Nat Rev Immunol.* 2004;4:978-988.
207. Strachan DP. Hay fever, hygiene, and household size. *Bmj.* 1989;299:1259-1260.
208. Stene LC, Nafstad P. Relation between occurrence of type 1 diabetes and asthma. *Lancet.* 2001;357:607-608.
209. Noverr MC, Huffnagle GB. The 'microflora hypothesis' of allergic diseases. *Clin Exp Allergy.* 2005;35:1511-1520.
210. Fallon PG, Mangan NE. Suppression of TH2-type allergic reactions by helminth infection. *Nat Rev Immunol.* 2007;7:220-230.
211. Viglietta V, Baecher-Allan C, Weiner HL, Hafler DA. Loss of functional suppression by CD4+CD25+ regulatory T cells in patients with multiple sclerosis. *J Exp Med.* 2004;199:971-979.
212. Arif S, Tree TI, Astill TP, et al. Autoreactive T cell responses show proinflammatory polarization in diabetes but a regulatory phenotype in health. *J Clin Invest.* 2004;113:451-463.
213. Karlsson MR, Rugtveit J, Brandtzaeg P. Allergen-responsive CD4+CD25+ regulatory T cells in children who have outgrown cow's milk allergy. *J Exp Med.* 2004;199:1679-1688.
214. Bjorksten B, Naaber P, Sepp E, Mikelsaar M. The intestinal microflora in allergic Estonian and Swedish 2-year-old children. *Clin Exp Allergy.* 1999;29:342-346.
215. Bjorksten B, Sepp E, Julge K, Voor T, Mikelsaar M. Allergy development and the intestinal microflora during the first year of life. *J Allergy Clin Immunol.* 2001;108:516-520.
216. Kalliomaki M, Kirjavainen P, Eerola E, Kero P, Salminen S, Isolauri E. Distinct patterns of neonatal gut microflora in infants in whom atopy was and was not developing. *J Allergy Clin Immunol.* 2001;107:129-134.
217. Di Giacinto C, Marinaro M, Sanchez M, Strober W, Boirivant M. Probiotics ameliorate recurrent Th1-mediated murine colitis by inducing IL-10 and IL-10-dependent TGF-beta-bearing regulatory cells. *J Immunol.* 2005;174:3237-3246.
218. Geier MS, Butler RN, Howarth GS. Inflammatory bowel disease: current insights into pathogenesis and new therapeutic options; probiotics, prebiotics and synbiotics. *Int J Food Microbiol.* 2007;115:1-11.
219. Del Giudice MM, Rocco A, Capristo C. Probiotics in the atopic march: highlights and new insights. *Dig Liver Dis.* 2006;38 Suppl 2:S288-290.
220. Summers RW, Elliott DE, Urban JF, Jr., Thompson R, Weinstock JV. Trichuris suis therapy in Crohn's disease. *Gut.* 2005;54:87-90.

221. Summers RW, Elliott DE, Urban JF, Jr., Thompson RA, Weinstock JV. Trichuris suis therapy for active ulcerative colitis: a randomized controlled trial. *Gastroenterology.* 2005;128:825-832.
222. Cooper PJ, Chico ME, Rodrigues LC, et al. Reduced risk of atopy among school-age children infected with geohelminth parasites in a rural area of the tropics. *J Allergy Clin Immunol.* 2003;111:995-1000.
223. Scrivener S, Yemaneberhan H, Zebenigus M, et al. Independent effects of intestinal parasite infection and domestic allergen exposure on risk of wheeze in Ethiopia: a nested case-control study. *Lancet.* 2001;358:1493-1499.
224. van den Biggelaar AH, Rodrigues LC, van Ree R, et al. Long-term treatment of intestinal helminths increases mite skin-test reactivity in Gabonese schoolchildren. *J Infect Dis.* 2004;189:892-900.
225. Wilson MS, Taylor MD, Balic A, Finney CA, Lamb JR, Maizels RM. Suppression of allergic airway inflammation by helminth-induced regulatory T cells. *J Exp Med.* 2005;202:1199-1212.
226. McKee AS, Pearce EJ. CD25+CD4+ cells contribute to Th2 polarization during helminth infection by suppressing Th1 response development. *J Immunol.* 2004;173:1224-1231.
227. Westall FC. Molecular mimicry revisited: gut bacteria and multiple sclerosis. *J Clin Microbiol.* 2006;44:2099-2104.
228. Scarpa R, Manguso F, D'Arienzo A, et al. Microscopic inflammatory changes in colon of patients with both active psoriasis and psoriatic arthritis without bowel symptoms. *J Rheumatol.* 2000;27:1241-1246.
229. Caserta L, de Magistris L, Secondulfo M, et al. Assessment of intestinal permeability and orocecal transit time in patients with systemic sclerosis: analysis of relationships with epidemiologic and clinical parameters. *Rheumatol Int.* 2003;23:226-230.
230. Kovacs T, Kun L, Schmelczer M, Wagner L, Davin JC, Nagy J. Do intestinal hyperpermeability and the related food antigens play a role in the progression of IgA nephropathy? I. Study of intestinal permeability. *Am J Nephrol.* 1996;16:500-505.
231. Collin P, Syrjanen J, Partanen J, Pasternack A, Kaukinen K, Mustonen J. Celiac disease and HLA DQ in patients with IgA nephropathy. *Am J Gastroenterol.* 2002;97:2572-2576.
232. Feld JJ, Meddings J, Heathcote EJ. Abnormal intestinal permeability in primary biliary cirrhosis. *Dig Dis Sci.* 2006;51:1607-1613.
233. Eerola E, Mottonen T, Hannonen P, et al. Intestinal flora in early rheumatoid arthritis. *Br J Rheumatol.* 1994;33:1030-1038.
234. Bosi E, Molteni L, Radaelli MG, et al. Increased intestinal permeability precedes clinical onset of type 1 diabetes. *Diabetologia.* 2006;49:2824-2827.
235. Schwartz RF, Neu J, Schatz D, Atkinson MA, Wasserfall C. Comment on: Brugman S et al. (2006) Antibiotic treatment partially protects against type 1 diabetes in the Bio-Breeding diabetes-prone rat. Is the gut flora involved in the development of type 1 diabetes? Diabetologia 49:2105-2108. *Diabetologia.* 2007;50:220-221.
236. Turvey SE. Atopic diseases of childhood. *Curr Opin Pediatr.* 2001;13:487-495.
237. Johansson SG, Hourihane JO, Bousquet J, et al. A revised nomenclature for allergy. An EAACI position statement from the EAACI nomenclature task force. *Allergy.* 2001;56:813-824.
238. O'Connell EJ. The burden of atopy and asthma in children. *Allergy.* 2004;59 Suppl 78:7-11.
239. Eder W, Ege MJ, von Mutius E. The asthma epidemic. *N Engl J Med.* 2006;355:2226-2235.
240. Bjorksten B. Effects of intestinal microflora and the environment on the development of asthma and allergy. *Springer Semin Immunopathol.* 2004;25:257-270.
241. Alm JS, Swartz J, Bjorksten B, et al. An anthroposophic lifestyle and intestinal microflora in infancy. *Pediatr Allergy Immunol.* 2002;13:402-411.
242. Rosenfeldt V, Benfeldt E, Nielsen SD, et al. Effect of probiotic Lactobacillus strains in children with atopic dermatitis. *J Allergy Clin Immunol.* 2003;111:389-395.
243. Isolauri E, Arvola T, Sutas Y, Moilanen E, Salminen S. Probiotics in the management of atopic eczema. *Clin Exp Allergy.* 2000;30:1604-1610.
244. Ciprandi G, Vizzaccaro A, Cirillo I, Tosca MA. Bacillus clausii effects in children with allergic rhinitis. *Allergy.* 2005;60:702-703.
245. Giovannini M, Agostoni C, Riva E, et al. A randomized prospective double blind controlled trial on effects of long-term consumption of fermented milk containing Lactobacillus casei in pre-school children with allergic asthma and/or rhinitis. *Pediatr Res.* 2007;62:215-220.
246. Lodinova-Zadnikova R, Cukrowska B, Tlaskalova-Hogenova H. Oral administration of probiotic Escherichia coli after birth reduces frequency of allergies and repeated infections later in life (after 10 and 20 years). *Int Arch Allergy Immunol.* 2003;131:209-211.
247. Rautava S, Kalliomaki M, Isolauri E. Probiotics during pregnancy and breast-feeding might confer immunomodulatory protection against atopic disease in the infant. *J Allergy Clin Immunol.* 2002;109:119-121.
248. Benard A, Desreumeaux P, Huglo D, Hoorelbeke A, Tonnel AB, Wallaert B. Increased intestinal permeability in bronchial asthma. *J Allergy Clin Immunol.* 1996;97:1173-1178.
249. Hijazi Z, Molla AM, Al-Habashi H, Muawad WM, Molla AM, Sharma PN. Intestinal permeability is increased in bronchial asthma. *Arch Dis Child.* 2004;89:227-229.
250. Pike MG, Heddle RJ, Boulton P, Turner MW, Atherton DJ. Increased intestinal permeability in atopic eczema. *J Invest Dermatol.* 1986;86:101-104.
251. Rosenfeldt V, Benfeldt E, Valerius NH, Paerregaard A, Michaelsen KF. Effect of probiotics on gastrointestinal symptoms and small intestinal permeability in children with atopic dermatitis. *J Pediatr.* 2004;145:612-616.
252. Oien T, Storro O, Johnsen R. Intestinal microbiota and its effect on the immune system--a nested case-cohort study on prevention of atopy among small children in Trondheim: the IMPACT study. *Contemp Clin Trials.* 2006;27:389-395.
253. Shinebaum R, Neumann VC, Cooke EM, Wright V. Comparison of faecal florae in patients with rheumatoid arthritis and controls. *Br J Rheumatol.* 1987;26:329-333.
254. Melief MJ, Hoijer MA, Van Paassen HC, Hazenberg MP. Presence of bacterial flora-derived antigen in synovial tissue macrophages and dendritic cells. *Br J Rheumatol.* 1995;34:1112-1116.
255. Mielants H, De Vos M, Goemaere S, et al. Intestinal mucosal permeability in inflammatory rheumatic diseases. II. Role of disease. *J Rheumatol.* 1991;18:394-400.
256. Smith MD, Gibson RA, Brooks PM. Abnormal bowel permeability in ankylosing spondylitis and rheumatoid arthritis. *J Rheumatol.* 1985;12:299-305.
257. Fagiolo U, Paganelli R, Ossi E, et al. Intestinal permeability and antigen absorption in rheumatoid arthritis. Effects of acetylsalicylic acid and sodium chromoglycate. *Int Arch Allergy Appl Immunol.* 1989;89:98-102.
258. Bjarnason I, Williams P, So A, et al. Intestinal permeability and inflammation in rheumatoid arthritis: effects of non-steroidal anti-inflammatory drugs. *Lancet.* 1984;2:1171-1174.
259. Dearlove SM, Barr K, Neumann V, et al. The effect of non-steroidal anti-inflammatory drugs on faecal flora and bacterial antibody levels in rheumatoid arthritis. *Br J Rheumatol.* 1992;31:443-447.

260. Hirata D, Hirai I, Iwamoto M, et al. Preferential binding with Escherichia coli hsp60 of antibodies prevalent in sera from patients with rheumatoid arthritis. *Clin Immunol Immunopathol.* 1997;82:141-148.
261. Maki-Ikola O, Hallgren R, Kanerud L, Feltelius N, Knutsson L, Granfors K. Enhanced jejunal production of antibodies to Klebsiella and other Enterobacteria in patients with ankylosing spondylitis and rheumatoid arthritis. *Ann Rheum Dis.* 1997;56:421-425.
262. Chou CT, Uksila J, Toivanen P. Enterobacterial antibodies in Chinese patients with rheumatoid arthritis and ankylosing spondylitis. *Clin Exp Rheumatol.* 1998;16:161-164.
263. Toivanen P. From reactive arthritis to rheumatoid arthritis. *J Autoimmun.* 2001;16:369-371.
264. Stone M, Fortin PR, Pacheco-Tena C, Inman RD. Should tetracycline treatment be used more extensively for rheumatoid arthritis? Metaanalysis demonstrates clinical benefit with reduction in disease activity. *J Rheumatol.* 2003;30:2112-2122.
265. Case JP. Old and new drugs used in rheumatoid arthritis: a historical perspective. Part 2: the newer drugs and drug strategies. *Am J Ther.* 2001;8:163-179.
266. Galland L. Minocycline and rheumatoid arthritis revisited. *Ann Intern Med.* 1995;123:392-393.
267. Hafstrom I, Ringertz B, Spangberg A, et al. A vegan diet free of gluten improves the signs and symptoms of rheumatoid arthritis: the effects on arthritis correlate with a reduction in antibodies to food antigens. *Rheumatology (Oxford).* 2001;40:1175-1179.
268. Peltonen R, Kjeldsen-Kragh J, Haugen M, et al. Changes of faecal flora in rheumatoid arthritis during fasting and one-year vegetarian diet. *Br J Rheumatol.* 1994;33:638-643.
269. Peltonen R, Nenonen M, Helve T, Hanninen O, Toivanen P, Eerola E. Faecal microbial flora and disease activity in rheumatoid arthritis during a vegan diet. *Br J Rheumatol.* 1997;36:64-68.
270. Toivanen P, Eerola E. A vegan diet changes the intestinal flora. *Rheumatology (Oxford).* 2002;41:950-951.
271. Hvatum M, Kanerud L, Hallgren R, Brandtzaeg P. The gut-joint axis: cross reactive food antibodies in rheumatoid arthritis. *Gut.* 2006;55:1240-1247.
272. Podas T, Nightingale JM, Oldham R, Roy S, Sheehan NJ, Mayberry JF. Is rheumatoid arthritis a disease that starts in the intestine? A pilot study comparing an elemental diet with oral prednisolone. *Postgrad Med J.* 2007;83:128-131.
273. Muller H, de Toledo FW, Resch KL. Fasting followed by vegetarian diet in patients with rheumatoid arthritis: a systematic review. *Scand J Rheumatol.* 2001;30:1-10.
274. Mankertz J, Schulzke JD. Altered permeability in inflammatory bowel disease: pathophysiology and clinical implications. *Curr Opin Gastroenterol.* 2007;23:379-383.
275. Fiasse R, Latinne D. Intestinal helminths: a clue explaining the low incidence of inflammatory bowel diseases in Subsaharan Africa? Potential benefits and hazards of helminth therapy. *Acta Gastroenterol Belg.* 2006;69:418-422.
276. Gillespie KM, Bain SC, Barnett AH, et al. The rising incidence of childhood type 1 diabetes and reduced contribution of high-risk HLA haplotypes. *Lancet.* 2004;364:1699-1700.
277. Brugman S, Klatter FA, Visser JT, et al. Antibiotic treatment partially protects against type 1 diabetes in the Bio-Breeding diabetes-prone rat. Is the gut flora involved in the development of type 1 diabetes? *Diabetologia.* 2006;49:2105-2108.
278. Calcinaro F, Dionisi S, Marinaro M, et al. Oral probiotic administration induces interleukin-10 production and prevents spontaneous autoimmune diabetes in the non-obese diabetic mouse. *Diabetologia.* 2005;48:1565-1575.
279. Ljungberg M, Korpela R, Ilonen J, Ludvigsson J, Vaarala O. Probiotics for the prevention of beta cell autoimmunity in children at genetic risk of type 1 diabetes--the PRODIA study. *Ann N Y Acad Sci.* 2006;1079:360-364.
280. Saunders KA, Raine T, Cooke A, Lawrence CE. Inhibition of autoimmune type 1 diabetes by gastrointestinal helminth infection. *Infect Immun.* 2007;75:397-407.
281. Sapone A, de Magistris L, Pietzak M, et al. Zonulin upregulation is associated with increased gut permeability in subjects with type 1 diabetes and their relatives. *Diabetes.* 2006;55:1443-1449.
282. Vaarala O. Is it dietary insulin? *Ann N Y Acad Sci.* 2006;1079:350-359.
283. Kimpimaki T, Erkkola M, Korhonen S, et al. Short-term exclusive breastfeeding predisposes young children with increased genetic risk of Type I diabetes to progressive beta-cell autoimmunity. *Diabetologia.* 2001;44:63-69.
284. Cavallo MG, Fava D, Monetini L, Barone F, Pozzilli P. Cell-mediated immune response to beta casein in recent-onset insulin-dependent diabetes: implications for disease pathogenesis. *Lancet.* 1996;348:926-928.
285. Rodemann JF, Dubberke ER, Reske KA, Seo da H, Stone CD. Incidence of Clostridium difficile infection in inflammatory bowel disease. *Clin Gastroenterol Hepatol.* 2007;5:339-344.

Chapter 3

Conventional Approaches to Treatment of Gastrointestinal and Systemic Diseases

In this chapter, we will provide an overview of conventional approaches to assessing and treating 4 conditions conventionally considered discrete disease entities: inflammatory bowel disease, irritable bowel syndrome, rheumatoid arthritis, and fibromyalgia. We will discuss how healthcare practitioners make the differential diagnosis between inflammatory bowel disease and irritable bowel syndrome and between rheumatoid arthritis and fibromyalgia, and we will present a brief overview of the different treatment approaches to these disorders, two of which are considered *organic* diseases, and two of which (irritable bowel syndrome and fibromyalgia) are considered *functional* diseases. We rely on recent comprehensive reviews for information about current conventional approaches to treatment of these complex disorders; we realize, however, that individual practitioners will have their own approaches.

In Chapter 4, we will introduce the concepts of antecedents, triggers, and mediators of disease as a different way to approach patients with these conditions, and finally in Chapter 5, we will present a functional medicine approach to evaluation and treatment of these difficult conditions.

Inflammatory Bowel Disease and Irritable Bowel Syndrome

Diagnosis

In patients presenting with symptoms suggestive of disturbances in the large bowel, including but not limited to abdominal discomfort, change in bowel habit, diarrhea, abdominal pain, distention, pain associated with defecation, passage of mucus or blood, and weight loss, 2 diagnoses that must be considered are inflammatory bowel disease (either ulcerative colitis or Crohn's disease) and irritable bowel syndrome. Inflammatory bowel disease is, as its name implies, a disease of the gastrointestinal tract characterized by inflammation that may occur in response to the normal microbial contents of the gut lumen.[1] In contrast, irritable bowel syndrome is generally considered one of a group of disorders grouped under the title *functional gastrointestinal disorders*,[2] in which "no specific biological marker, physiological abnormality, or anatomical defect has been discovered."[3] While several other possible diagnoses would obviously be considered in patients presenting with the symptoms listed above, inflammatory bowel disease and irritable bowel syndrome are, as discussed in Chapter 1, common disorders and would therefore be high on a healthcare practitioner's list of differential diagnoses. Various disease features and diagnostic criteria can facilitate the differential diagnosis between inflammatory bowel disease and irritable bowel syndrome, as well as to differentiate between various disease subcategories.[3-9]

Inflammatory bowel disease — Alarm or red flag features of organic, rather than functional, disease include weight loss, nocturnal awakenings with gastrointestinal symptoms, fever, bloody stool, recent onset of symptoms, onset of symptoms after age 50, recent use of antibiotics, family history of cancer or inflammatory bowel disease, the presence of an abdominal mass, occult blood in the stool, or enlarged lymph nodes.[3-5] These alarm features would lead the practitioner to consider inflammatory bowel disease rather than irritable bowel syndrome as a possible diagnosis.

Inflammatory bowel disease is largely a clinical diagnosis[1, 8] that depends on "the aggregate constellation of the clinical history, physical findings, and endoscopic, radiological, and histological features, as well as the results of routine laboratory tests."[1] Overt inflammation in the bowel is clearly a hallmark of the disease. Generally, a diagnosis of inflammatory bowel disease is made after other causes of colitis, including but not limited to infections, microscopic colitis, diverticulitis, toxic colitis, and vasculitis, have been ruled out.[8] Further categorization into Crohn's disease or ulcerative colitis categories, based on clinical picture, endoscopic findings, and histological findings, follows the initial diagnosis.[1, 8] Ulcerative colitis is characterized by the presence of nontransmural inflammation restricted to the colon.[8] Crohn's disease is characterized by the presence of transmural inflammation that can affect the entire gastrointestinal tract from the mouth to the anus.[8] Clear differentiation into one or other disease category is often difficult, however,[9] and in up to 10% of patients with disease limited to the colon, accurate separation is not possible.[1]

Irritable bowel syndrome — Clinical history is the main tool used to diagnose irritable bowel syndrome.[3] In 1994, Drossman et al introduced a formal system for classification and diagnosis of functional gastrointestinal disorders.[10] The diagnostic criteria are continually being updated; currently, Rome III criteria are used for diagnostic and research purposes.[7] The Rome III criteria for a diagnosis of irritable bowel syndrome are "recurrent abdominal pain or discomfort at least 3 days per month in the past 3 months associated with two or more of the following: improvement with defecation; onset with change of frequency of stool; and onset associated with a change in the form and appearance of the stool." The criteria must be fulfilled for at least the past 3 months, with symptom onset at least 6 months before diagnosis.[7] Although these criteria are useful for research purposes, their applicability in clinical practice has been questioned by several authors,[4, 11] and the diagnosis of irritable bowel syndrome is often difficult to make with confidence[12]; the diagnosis is often made intuitively rather than by following specific diagnostic criteria.[11, 13] Extensive diagnostic testing may be undertaken in the presence of the alarm features discussed above.[4, 5]

Clinical Pearl:

Intestinal protozoan infestation is a relatively common occurrence in patients with a diagnosis of irritable bowel syndrome or ulcerative colitis. All patients with these diagnoses should be tested for parasites and treated appropriately. The likelihood of protozoan infection is greatest in those with a recent acute onset or an acute exacerbation of a previously stable condition. Foreign travel is not needed for protozoan infestation to occur.

Treatment

Based on whether the diagnosis is irritable bowel syndrome or inflammatory bowel disease, practitioners will employ very different treatments.

Inflammatory bowel disease — Treatment of inflammatory bowel disease consists of certain established therapies, as well as a number of newer agents, all of which are designed to suppress inflammation.[8] Treatment of active disease and maintenance of remission have been described as "daunting and challenging tasks."[14] Here, we will concentrate on established therapies, which include 5-aminosalicylic acid compounds, corticosteroids, immunosuppressive agents, and the newer biologic anti-TNF agents.[1, 8] Initial treatment depends on the severity of the disease and the location in the gastrointestinal tract.

The 5-aminosalicylic acid-based compounds, such as mesalamine and sulfasalazine, are considered mainstays of treatment for mild to moderately active ulcerative colitis or Crohn's disease,[1] although first-line treatment for patients with Crohn's disease is controversial because mesalamine is not always effective.[8] Mesalazine is generally well-tolerated, but the use of sulfasalazine is limited by the frequent appearance of secretory diarrhea at higher doses.[15]

Oral corticosteroids are the second line of treatment and are commonly used when 5-aminosalicylates fail to induce remission.[1, 8] A population study showed that 34% of patients with ulcerative colitis and 44% of patients with Crohn's disease needed treatment with corticosteroids to achieve remission[16]; notably, after 1 year, 51% of patients with ulcerative colitis and 68% of patients with Crohn's disease were either steroid-dependent or required surgery.[16] For patients in whom oral corticosteroids are not effective, intravenous corticosteroids may be needed.[8] Corticosteroids have been described as the "Dr. Jekyll and Mr. Hyde" of inflammatory bowel disease therapy.[17] Despite their frequent success at inducing and maintaining remission, it has been pointed out that "no other commonly used therapy causes so many difficult and damaging treatment-related side effects."[17] The well-known side effects of steroid therapy include metabolic, dermatologic, ocular, neuropsychiatric, and immunologic disturbances.[17]

Table 3.1—Adverse Events with Corticosteroids[18]

- Early events—Cosmetic side effects (acne, moon facies, edema), sleep disturbance, mood disturbance, glucose intolerance, dyspepsia
- Events with prolonged use (usually > 12 weeks)—Posterior sublenticular cataracts, osteoporosis, osteonecrosis of the femoral head, myopathy, susceptibility to infections
- Events with withdrawal—Acute adrenal insufficiency, myalgias, malaise, arthralgias, increased intracranial pressure

For patients in whom the dose of corticosteroids cannot be tapered or discontinued, several immunosuppressive agents can be used, including azathioprine, mercaptopurine, methotrexate (for Crohn's disease), cyclosporine (for ulcerative colitis), and tacrolimus (for ulcerative colitis).[1, 8] Azathioprine and mercaptopurine are generally the next line of treatment for both ulcerative colitis and Cohn's disease,[1] although data concerning their efficacy in ulcerative colitis is "sparse and inconsistent."[8] When used to maintain remission in patients with Crohn's disease, these drugs (methotrexate being a third option) may need to be continued indefinitely.[8] Cyclosporine and tacrolimus are used for patients with severe ulcerative colitis who do not respond to steroids, although there is insufficient data to determine which of these agents is more effective.[8] In patients with fistulizing Crohn's disease, antibiotics, in particular metronidazole, are widely used as first-line therapy[1, 8]; a recent meta-analysis of studies of metronidazole or other broad-spectrum antibiotics demonstrated improved clinical outcomes.[19]

As with corticosteroids, toxic effects frequently limit the use of azathioprine and mercaptopurine; these include a uniformly observed, dose-related suppression of bone marrow, as well as hepatic damage, pancreatitis, and a possible increased risk of lymphoma. Methotrexate may also cause interstitial pneumonitis.[1] Viral infections are common in patients treated with the immunosuppressive agents listed above; indeed, the most common cause of mortality associated with therapies used in inflammatory bowel disease is infection.[20]

In recent years, therapy with so-called biologic agents such as the anti-TNF antibody infliximab has become more widespread. Infliximab can be used in patients with either ulcerative colitis or Crohn's disease that is refractory to treatment with steroids and other immunosuppressive agents.[1, 8] Use of biologic agents has led to improved quality of life and fewer hospital admissions for many patients with inflammatory bowel disease.[1, 20] Nevertheless, these agents, which "interfere with key molecules in the human physiology,"[20] are still being used "with reluctance," in large part because of concerns about their safety.[1, 20] As with the immunosuppressive agents listed above, the most common cause of mortality associated with biologic therapies is infection.[20] While the use of immunosuppressive agents is often associated with viral infections such as cytomegalovirus and Epstein-Barr virus infections, use of anti-TNF agents such as infliximab is more commonly associated with mycobacterial infections (such as tuberculosis and histoplasmosis), as well as other opportunistic infections such as listeriosis, nocardiosis, and invasive aspergillosis.[20]

Table 3.2—Adverse Events with Biologic Agents[21]

- Increased risk of opportunistic infections, including tuberculosis
- Development of autoimmunity (antinuclear and anti-DNA antibodies)
- Infusion and injection site reactions
- Development of antibodies against therapies
- Neurological disorders such as optic neuritis, seizure, and new onset or exacerbation of central demyelinating disorders, including multiple sclerosis
- Congestive heart failure
- Lymphomas and other malignancies

In severe cases of inflammatory bowel disease with life-threatening complications or when medical management does not lead to improvement, elective or emergency surgery may be necessary. Indeed, 24% of patients with ulcerative colitis will have had a colectomy by 10 years after diagnosis.[8] The most common elective procedure used in patients with ulcerative colitis is total proctocolectomy with ileal J-pouch-anal anastomosis. Complications include the need for repeat surgery, pelvic sepsis, pouchitis, pouch failure, high stool frequency, fecal incontinence, and reduced fertility.[8] A 2005 meta-analysis of outcomes after ileal pouch anastomosis showed pouch failure in 6.8% of patients, pelvic sepsis in 9.5% of patients, and fecal incontinence in up to 17% (mild) of patients after 36.7 months of follow-up.[22] The presence of fistulizing Crohn's disease also frequently necessitates surgical intervention; after 20 years, most patients with Crohn's disease will require surgery.[8]

Both the rapid pace of the search for therapies (a 2002 review[1] lists 20 potential therapeutic agents for inflammatory bowel disease, and a 2007 review[8] lists 37 investigational therapies) and the high level of required surgical intervention highlight the relative lack of efficacy of many conventional treatments for inflammatory bowel disease. The authors of a recent review on Crohn's disease noted that "despite the fact that immunomodulators and infliximab are effective in maintaining clinical and endoscopic remission, there is little hard evidence at present that these therapies alter the natural history of the disease."[23]

Irritable bowel syndrome — The treatment of irritable bowel syndrome, which has been described as "notoriously unsatisfactory,"[4] differs dramatically from the treatment of inflammatory bowel disease. Whereas in inflammatory bowel disease, several potent anti-inflammatory and immunosuppressive drugs are used, treatment of irritable bowel syndrome relies heavily on nonspecific supportive therapies, aimed primarily at relieving symptoms; indeed, a *New England Journal of Medicine* review article suggests that a "rational approach to treating the irritable bowel syndrome uses the patient's symptoms as a guide."[24] Several clinical updates have discussed current treatment approaches to patients with irritable bowel syndrome.[3-5, 24] The American Gastroenterological Association, in a position statement released in 2002, divided therapies into the general treatment approach, medication directed at the predominant symptom, psychological treatments (psychotherapy, meditation, stress management, relaxation), and centrally acting medications.[25]

Patient education and reassurance, explanation about the disorder, and help with dietary and other lifestyle modifications are considered part of the general treatment approach.[3, 5, 24, 25] Establishing trust in the physician-patient relationship is considered essential.[24] Dietary modification is frequently advised for patients with irritable bowel syndrome,[4] although the role of this intervention has been described as uncertain.[3, 5] Foods that patients feel exacerbate symptoms can be excluded (and patients frequently undertake these modifications on their own); at least one study has found that food elimination based on IgG antibodies can reduce irritable bowel syndrome symptoms.[26] Fiber can be added to the diet, although there is evidence that insoluble fiber may actually worsen the condition by exacerbating bloating and pain.[4]

In terms of pharmacological therapies, treatment is directed mainly at alleviating the predominant symptoms of pain, diarrhea, or constipation.[3, 24, 25] When pain is the predominant symptom, anticholinergic agents (antispasmodics) are commonly used.[3, 24] In addition, tricyclic antidepressants[3, 4, 25] and selective serotonin reuptake inhibitors[3, 24, 25] may be prescribed for pain, as well as comorbid psychiatric symptoms. Serotonin receptor antagonists have also been used for pain-predominant irritable bowel syndrome, although the results have been described as disappointing.[24] The issue of efficacy is now somewhat moot, as tegaserod, a 5-HT_4 antagonist, was withdrawn from the market in 2007 following reports of increased adverse cardiovascular events,[3] and alosetron, a 5-HT_3 receptor antagonist, can be used only if prescribing physicians register with the manufacturer because of concerns about gastrointestinal toxicity.[3] When diarrhea is the predominant symptom, antidiarrheal agents such as loperamide or diphenoxylate are commonly prescribed, and antibiotics can be prescribed in refractory cases; alosetron (with the restrictions noted above) is also used.[3, 24, 25] And when constipation is predominant, osmotic laxatives are used.[3, 24]

The issue of side effects of pharmacological agents is certainly important in patients with irritable bowel syndrome (for example, side effects of the tricyclic antidepressants such as dry mouth, sedation, and dry eyes limit their use[24]); however, lack of efficacy of current treatments appears to be a more pressing issue. The authors of a Cochrane review[27] of 40 studies concluded that the evidence for efficacy of drug therapies is weak and that there is no clear evidence of benefit for antidepressants or bulking agents. It has also been noted that true drug effects are smaller than the placebo effect in most randomized trials.[5] And the authors of another recent study concluded that "there are significant unmet needs including lack of familiarity with irritable bowel syndrome, difficulties in diagnosis and lack of effective treatments for the multiple symptoms of the disorder."[13]

Rheumatoid Arthritis and Fibromyalgia

In patients presenting with symptoms suggestive of musculoskeletal dysfunction such as pain and stiffness, diagnoses that need to be considered include rheumatoid arthritis and fibromyalgia. Like inflammatory bowel disease and irritable bowel syndrome, these conditions are often separated into functional and organic categories of disease, and similar to patients with the bowel disturbances described above, many people with these musculoskeletal disorders are unable to find relief using conventional treatment.

Diagnosis

Rheumatoid arthritis — Rheumatoid arthritis has been described as the "paradigmatic immune-mediated inflammatory arthropathy."[28] The disease affects about 1% of the population worldwide. Although the definition is sometimes imprecise,[29] the disease is usually diagnosed based on the presence of a symmetrical destructive arthritis that is often associated with the presence in the blood of rheumatoid factor (an antibody directed against IgG), anti-cyclic citrullinated peptide antibodies, or several other autoantibodies.[29, 30] Diagnosis of early disease can be challenging. The criteria developed by the American College of Rheumatology[31] (the presence of morning stiffness, arthritis of 3 or more joint areas, symmetrical arthritis, serum rheumatoid factor, and radiographic changes) have a sensitivity of only 40% to 60% in patients with early rheumatoid arthritis in whom there may be no radiographic changes.[32] In addition, synovitis is particularly difficult to diagnose by physical examination, and inflammatory polyarthritis has a large differential diagnosis which includes post-viral arthralgia, other autoimmune diseases, and functional peripheral pain disorders such as fibromyalgia.[32, 33]

Clinical Pearl:

Patients with autoimmune disorders often suffer from impairment of the hypothalamic-pituitary-adrenal (HPA) axis, which has been documented in untreated patients but can be exacerbated by the use of glucocorticoids. HPA axis defects can be demonstrated by measurement of salivary or urinary free cortisol or serum DHEA-S or by a low-dose ACTH stimulation test. Correction or compensation for these defects may positively affect the course of the illness.

Fibromyalgia — Fibromyalgia is a far more common and poorly understood disorder than rheumatoid arthritis, affecting up to 12% of the population, and the condition has a complex array of symptoms and poor treatment outcome.[34, 35] The diagnosis of fibromyalgia is difficult. In 1990 the American College of Rheumatology published a list of diagnostic criteria for fibromyalgia, including a history of widespread pain (defined as bilateral, upper and lower body, and spine) and the presence of excessive tenderness when applying pressure to 11 of 18 specific muscle-tendon sites.[36] As with the criteria discussed above for irritable bowel syndrome, some authors do not believe that these criteria are useful for diagnosing fibromyalgia in clinical practice[33]; diagnosis is often made on the basis of clinical history and the absence of markers of other organic diseases such as rheumatoid arthritis, osteoarthritis, or other regional pain syndromes.[33, 35] The lack of unique pathophysiological characteristics and the overlap between fibromyalgia and other disorders such as chronic fatigue syndrome, irritable bowel syndrome, mood disturbances, and chronic muscular headaches make both diagnosis and management extremely difficult[35]; indeed, a recent narrative review on the topic noted that "no consensus exists on the syndrome's cause, its treatment, or even whether it merits consideration as a distinct clinical entity."[37]

Treatment

Similar to the differences between therapies for patients diagnosed with either inflammatory bowel disease or irritable bowel syndrome, treatment strategies vary greatly between rheumatoid arthritis and fibromyalgia.

Rheumatoid arthritis—Guidelines for the management of rheumatoid arthritis were created by the American College of Rheumatology Subcommittee on Rheumatoid Arthritis and published in 2002.[38] Noting that "the ultimate goals in managing [rheumatoid arthritis] are to prevent or control joint damage, prevent loss of function, and decrease pain," these guidelines recommend nonsteroidal anti-inflammatory drugs (NSAIDs) as initial treatment. These drugs are often effective at reducing pain in all stages of rheumatoid arthritis; however, they do not have any beneficial effect on disease progression.[29, 38] Indeed, their detrimental effects on gastrointestinal permeability, with the associated increase in antigen presentation to the gut immune system (discussed in Chapter 2), may mean that they contribute to the progression and persistence of disease even as they control pain. In addition to NSAIDs, local (intra-articular) or systemic steroids are frequently used. They appear to be effective in the short term in relieving signs and symptoms of disease, but the well-known side effects limit their long-term use.[28, 29]

Clinical Pearl:

Dietary supplements may offer protection against NSAID or aspirin enteropathy. L-glutamine[39] (7 g three times per day) and bovine colustrum[40] (125 mL three times per day) have each been shown to prevent the increase in small bowel permeability induced by indomethacin. Deglycyrrhizinated licorice (DGL, 325 mg three times per day) prevents aspirin-induced fecal blood loss. If your patients cannot avoid using these drugs, consider adding these supplements.

Disease-modifying antirheumatic drugs appear to slow progression of disease. Since the publication of the 2002 American College of Rheumatology guidelines, more emphasis has been placed on early introduction of disease-modifying drugs in an attempt to stave off joint damage, since progression of disease is often highest during the first 2 years after onset.[29] Several antirheumatic drugs are often used in combination. Methotrexate is considered the "anchor" disease-modifying drug[29] while others include hydroxychloroquine, sulfasalazine, leflunomide, and the newer biologic agents (discussed below).[38] All have significant side effects, including nausea, vomiting, abnormalities in liver function tests, pulmonary fibrosis (methotrexate), macular damage (hydroxychloroquine), and bone marrow depression (sulfasalazine and methotrexate).[38]

Biologic agents recommended for use in the 2002 guidelines include etanercept and infliximab (both anti-TNF agents).[38] Since then, a number of other biologic agents have been developed, including adalimumab (an anti-TNF agent), anakinra (an IL-1 receptor antagonist), rituximab (an anti-CD20 antibody), and abatacept (which blocks activation of T cells).[41] The side effects of these TNF antagonists have been discussed above in the section dealing with inflammatory bowel disease.

Tetracyclines have also been used to treat rheumatoid arthritis and are listed in the 2002 guidelines as disease-modifying drugs (with the qualifying statement that "further research is necessary to define the exact role of tetracyclines in the treatment of [rheumatoid arthritis]."[38] A 2003 meta-analysis of several trials concluded that tetracyclines, in particular minocycline, were associated with a significant reduction in disease activity[42]; the fact that they are not mentioned in 2 treatment strategy reviews[29, 43] published in 2007 suggests that they are not in common use in clinical practice.

Table 3.3—Toxicities of Drugs Used to Treat Rheumatoid Arthritis[38]

Drug/Category	Toxicities Requiring Monitoring
Salicylates; NSAIDs	Gastrointestinal ulceration and bleeding
Hydroxychloroquine	Macular damage
Sulfasalazine	Myelosuppression
Methotrexate	Myelosuppression, hepatic fibrosis, cirrhosis, pulmonary infiltrates or fibrosis
Leflunomide	Diarrhea, alopecia, rash, headache, theoretical risk of immunosuppression infection
Etanercept	Acute or chronic infection
Infliximab plus methotrexate	Acute or chronic infections, plus see methotrexate above
Azathioprine	Myelosuppression, hepatoxicity, lymphoproliferative disorders
D-penicillamine	Myelosuppression, proteinuria
Gold, intramuscular or oral	Myelosuppression, proteinuria
Minocycline	Hyperpigmentation, dizziness, vaginal yeast infections
Cyclosporine	Renal insufficiency, anemia, hypertension
Glucocorticoids	Hypertension, hyperglycemia, osteoporosis
Staphylococcal protein A immunoadsorption	Anemia, hypotension during procedure

Despite increased use of biologic agents and other disease-modifying drugs in rheumatoid arthritis, a recent review of more than 18,000 patients with rheumatoid arthritis, undertaken by the National Data Bank for Rheumatic Diseases, found not only that "remission remains uncommon in [rheumatoid arthritis]" but also that "the prevalence of new remission in community practice is substantially lower than noted in published trials of biologic therapy."[44]

Fibromyalgia — As in irritable bowel syndrome, several non-pharmacological treatments are used to treat patients with fibromyalgia. Intensive patient education about the (poorly understood) nature of the disorder seems to have a beneficial effect on symptoms and quality of life.[35] Exercise, both strength training and aerobic, has also been shown to be beneficial.[34, 35] Cognitive-behavioral therapy has been used over the past 2 decades; the author of a recent review[45] concluded that this therapy, as a single treatment modality, does not appear to provide any therapeutic advantage over education or exercise programs and suggested that further research is needed. Acupuncture is also used, although studies regarding its efficacy are inconclusive.[46]

A clue as to how difficult this disorder is to treat can be gleaned from the fact that only one drug (pregabalin) is currently approved by the FDA to treat fibromyalgia.[47] Thus, pharmacological management largely relies on drugs that are approved for other disorders. The author of a recent review noted that "drugs remain the primary treatment option for fibromyalgia" and that "the tricyclic antidepressants and their analogs are the drugs of choice."[34] Another researcher pointed out that "market surveys suggest that the no. 1 class of drugs currently used to treat fibromyalgia in the United States is NSAIDs, whereas opioids are no. 3 or 4, even though there is no evidence that either of these classes of drugs work in fibromyalgia."[33] And a recent survey of more than 2500 people with fibromyalgia revealed that the drugs most commonly used were acetaminophen, ibuprofen, naproxen, cyclobenzaprine (a tricyclic antidepressant), amitriptyline (a tricyclic antidepressant), and aspirin.[48]

Several different families of centrally acting drugs have been used for patients with fibromyalgia in clinical trials, although how frequently they are used in clinical practice is unclear. Tricyclic antidepressants such as amitriptyline and cyclobenzaprine have been used with good effect in several studies, although the trials have all been of short duration and there is no data on long-term use of tricyclics in patients with fibromyalgia. Improvement has been found to be mild for fatigue and moderate for pain, sleep, and overall well-being. Even at the low doses used, side effects such as dry mouth, constipation, fluid retention, weight gain, grogginess, and difficulty concentrating are common with tricyclic antidepressants.[49]

Serotonin reuptake inhibitors such as fluoxetine have also been used in clinical trials, although the results have been somewhat inconsistent.[49] More recently, dual (serotonin and norepinephrine) reuptake inhibitors such as duloxetine and milnacipran (currently approved for treatment of depression) have been used in clinical trials. Improvements in pain and overall function have been reported; side effects such as difficulty sleeping, oral dryness, and constipation, however, are common.[34, 49]

The anticonvulsant pregabalin, approved for use in fibromyalgia in June 2007,[47] has been found when used at high doses to improve pain, sleep, fatigue, and quality of life.[34] Whether it has moved into mainstream treatment at this time is uncertain. The most common side effects of pregabalin include dizziness and sleepiness, blurry vision, weight gain, trouble concentrating, swelling of the hands and feet, and dry mouth. Rarely, allergic reactions can occur.[47]

Although analgesics are commonly used to treat fibromyalgia, the only one that has been reported to be effective is tramadol, a novel analgesic that has some activity at μ receptors and also acts centrally to inhibit reuptake of serotonin and norepinephrine; it has been shown to reduce pain, alone or in combination with acetaminophen, but not the number of tender points.[49] The drug, which is probably not widely used in clinical practice for patients with fibromyalgia, has several side effects including seizures and serotonin syndrome (when it is used in combination with other drugs that affect serotonin reuptake); there is also concern regarding the risk of abuse.[49] As with all the conditions discussed in this chapter, research into pharmacological agents, including pindolol (a β-blocker), pramipexole (a dopamine agonist), gabapentin (an $\alpha_2 \delta$ ligand), human growth hormone, dehydroepiandrosterone, and 5-hydroxytryptophan, continues apace,[34, 49] again speaking to the relative lack of efficacy of current treatment options.

Summary

The basic method of the conventional approach to complex, chronic disease involves a process of differential diagnosis to define which disease is present; the function of diagnostic testing is largely to aid the process so that treatment appropriate to the assigned disease can be initiated. The conventional approach to treatment concentrates largely on pharmacological suppression of symptoms and inflammation. Despite continued research and development of drug therapies for all 4 conditions discussed in this chapter, many patients remain disabled because of lack of efficacy of available treatments, drug side effects, or uncontrolled disease.

References

1. Podolsky DK. Inflammatory bowel disease. *N Engl J Med.* 2002;347:417-429.
2. Corazziari E. Definition and epidemiology of functional gastrointestinal disorders. *Best Pract Res Clin Gastroenterol.* 2004;18:613-631.
3. Wilson JF. In the clinic. Irritable bowel syndrome. *Ann Intern Med.* 2007;147:ITC7-1-ITC7-16.
4. Agrawal A, Whorwell PJ. Irritable bowel syndrome: diagnosis and management. *Bmj.* 2006;332:280-283.
5. Spiller R. Clinical update: irritable bowel syndrome. *Lancet.* 2007;369:1586-1588.
6. Drossman DA. The functional gastrointestinal disorders and the Rome II process. *Gut.* 1999;45 Suppl 2:II1-5.
7. Drossman DA, Dumitrascu DL. Rome III: New standard for functional gastrointestinal disorders. *J Gastrointestin Liver Dis.* 2006;15:237-241.
8. Baumgart DC, Sandborn WJ. Inflammatory bowel disease: clinical aspects and established and evolving therapies. *Lancet.* 2007;369:1641-1657.
9. Bousvaros A, Antonioli DA, Colletti RB, et al. Differentiating ulcerative colitis from Crohn disease in children and young adults: report of a working group of the North American Society for Pediatric Gastroenterology, Hepatology, and Nutrition and the Crohn's and Colitis Foundation of America. *J Pediatr Gastroenterol Nutr.* 2007;44:653-674.

10. Drossman DA RJ, Talley NJ, Corazziari E, Thompson WG, Whitehead WE. *Functional Gastrointestinal Disorders*. Boston: Little Brown; 1994.
11. Vandvik PO, Aabakken L, Farup PG. Diagnosing irritable bowel syndrome: poor agreement between general practitioners and the Rome II criteria. *Scand J Gastroenterol*. 2004;39:448-453.
12. Longstreth GF. Definition and classification of irritable bowel syndrome: current consensus and controversies. *Gastroenterol Clin North Am*. 2005;34:173-187.
13. Quigley EM, Bytzer P, Jones R, Mearin F. Irritable bowel syndrome: the burden and unmet needs in Europe. *Dig Liver Dis*. 2006;38:717-723.
14. Tung JK, Warner AS. Colonic inflammatory bowel disease. Medical therapies for colonic Crohn's disease and ulcerative colitis. *Postgrad Med*. 2002;112:45-48, 51.
15. Hanauer SB. Review article: high-dose aminosalicylates to induce and maintain remissions in ulcerative colitis. *Aliment Pharmacol Ther*. 2006;24 Suppl 3:37-40.
16. Faubion WA, Jr., Loftus EV, Jr., Harmsen WS, Zinsmeister AR, Sandborn WJ. The natural history of corticosteroid therapy for inflammatory bowel disease: a population-based study. *Gastroenterology*. 2001;121:255-260.
17. Katz JA. Treatment of inflammatory bowel disease with corticosteroids. *Gastroenterol Clin North Am*. 2004;33:171-189, vii.
18. Lichtenstein GR, Abreu MT, Cohen R, Tremaine W. American Gastroenterological Association Institute technical review on corticosteroids, immunomodulators, and infliximab in inflammatory bowel disease. *Gastroenterology*. 2006;130:940-987.
19. Rahimi R, Nikfar S, Rezaie A, Abdollahi M. A meta-analysis of broad-spectrum antibiotic therapy in patients with active Crohn's disease. *Clin Ther*. 2006;28:1983-1988.
20. D'Haens G. Risks and benefits of biologic therapy for inflammatory bowel diseases. *Gut*. 2007;56:725-732.
21. Clark M, Colombel JF, Feagan BC, et al. American gastroenterological association consensus development conference on the use of biologics in the treatment of inflammatory bowel disease, June 21-23, 2006. *Gastroenterology*. 2007;133:312-339.
22. Hueting WE, Buskens E, van der Tweel I, Gooszen HG, van Laarhoven CJ. Results and complications after ileal pouch anal anastomosis: a meta-analysis of 43 observational studies comprising 9,317 patients. *Dig Surg*. 2005;22:69-79.
23. Vermeire S, van Assche G, Rutgeerts P. Review article: Altering the natural history of Crohn's disease--evidence for and against current therapies. *Aliment Pharmacol Ther*. 2007;25:3-12.
24. Horwitz BJ, Fisher RS. The irritable bowel syndrome. *N Engl J Med*. 2001;344:1846-1850.
25. American Gastroenterological Association medical position statement: irritable bowel syndrome. *Gastroenterology*. 2002;123:2105-2107.
26. Atkinson W, Sheldon TA, Shaath N, Whorwell PJ. Food elimination based on IgG antibodies in irritable bowel syndrome: a randomised controlled trial. *Gut*. 2004;53:1459-1464.
27. Quartero AO, Meineche-Schmidt V, Muris J, Rubin G, de Wit N. Bulking agents, antispasmodic and antidepressant medication for the treatment of irritable bowel syndrome. *Cochrane Database Syst Rev*. 2005:CD003460.
28. Case JP. Old and new drugs used in rheumatoid arthritis: a historical perspective. Part 1: the older drugs. *Am J Ther*. 2001;8:123-143.
29. Combe B. Early rheumatoid arthritis: strategies for prevention and management. *Best Pract Res Clin Rheumatol*. 2007;21:27-42.
30. Nishimura K, Sugiyama D, Kogata Y, et al. Meta-analysis: diagnostic accuracy of anti-cyclic citrullinated peptide antibody and rheumatoid factor for rheumatoid arthritis. *Ann Intern Med*. 2007;146:797-808.
31. Arnett FC, Edworthy SM, Bloch DA, et al. The American Rheumatism Association 1987 revised criteria for the classification of rheumatoid arthritis. *Arthritis Rheum*. 1988;31:315-324.
32. Cannella AC, O'Dell JR. Early rheumatoid arthritis: pitfalls in diagnosis and review of recent clinical trials. *Drugs*. 2006;66:1319-1337.
33. Clauw DJ. Fibromyalgia: update on mechanisms and management. *J Clin Rheumatol*. 2007;13:102-109.
34. Rooks DS. Fibromyalgia treatment update. *Curr Opin Rheumatol*. 2007;19:111-117.
35. Goldenberg DL, Burckhardt C, Crofford L. Management of fibromyalgia syndrome. *Jama*. 2004;292:2388-2395.
36. Wolfe F, Smythe HA, Yunus MB, et al. The American College of Rheumatology 1990 Criteria for the Classification of Fibromyalgia. Report of the Multicenter Criteria Committee. *Arthritis Rheum*. 1990;33:160-172.
37. Abeles AM, Pillinger MH, Solitar BM, Abeles M. Narrative review: the pathophysiology of fibromyalgia. *Ann Intern Med*. 2007;146:726-734.
38. Guidelines for the management of rheumatoid arthritis: 2002 Update. *Arthritis Rheum*. 2002;46:328-346.
39. Hond ED, Peeters M, Hiele M, Bulteel V, Ghoos Y, Rutgeerts P. Effect of glutamine on the intestinal permeability changes induced by indomethacin in humans. *Aliment Pharmacol Ther*. 1999;13:679-685.
40. Playford RJ, MacDonald CE, Calnan DP, et al. Co-administration of the health food supplement, bovine colostrum, reduces the acute non-steroidal anti-inflammatory drug-induced increase in intestinal permeability. *Clin Sci (Lond)*. 2001;100:627-633.
41. Lee SJ, Kavanaugh A. Biologic agents in rheumatology: safety considerations. *Rheum Dis Clin North Am*. 2006;32 Suppl 1:3-10.
42. Stone M, Fortin PR, Pacheco-Tena C, Inman RD. Should tetracycline treatment be used more extensively for rheumatoid arthritis? Metaanalysis demonstrates clinical benefit with reduction in disease activity. *J Rheumatol*. 2003;30:2112-2122.
43. Blom M, van Riel PL. Management of established rheumatoid arthritis with an emphasis on pharmacotherapy. *Best Pract Res Clin Rheumatol*. 2007;21:43-57.
44. Wolfe F, Rasker JJ, Boers M, Wells GA, Michaud K. Minimal disease activity, remission, and the long-term outcomes of rheumatoid arthritis. *Arthritis Rheum*. 2007;57:935-942.
45. Bennett R, Nelson D. Cognitive behavioral therapy for fibromyalgia. *Nat Clin Pract Rheumatol*. 2006;2:416-424.
46. Mayhew E, Ernst E. Acupuncture for fibromyalgia--a systematic review of randomized clinical trials. *Rheumatology (Oxford)*. 2007;46:801-804.
47. Living with Fibromyalgia, First Drug Approved. http://www.fda.gov/consumer/updates/fibromyalgia062107.html Accessed 9/10/2007.
48. Bennett RM, Jones J, Turk DC, Russell IJ, Matallana L. An internet survey of 2,596 people with fibromyalgia. *BMC Musculoskelet Disord*. 2007;8:27.
49. Goldenberg DL. Pharmacological treatment of fibromyalgia and other chronic musculoskeletal pain. *Best Pract Res Clin Rheumatol*. 2007;21:499-511.

Chapter 4

Antecedents, Triggers, and Mediators: A Functional Approach

The disease-centered approach described in Chapter 3 views each ailment as a discrete entity that can be classified according to an ICD code. Functional medicine, in contrast, views health and illness as a continuum in which all components of the human biological system interact dynamically with the environment. These interactions produce patterns that change over time in individuals. To manage the complexity inherent in this approach, functional medicine has adopted practical models for obtaining and evaluating clinical information that lead to individualized, patient-centered therapies. Chapters 4 and 5 will demonstrate the application of these models to the treatment of patients in whom gastrointestinal inflammation, permeability, and dysbiosis are important contributors to illnesses, including inflammatory bowel disease, irritable bowel syndrome, rheumatoid arthritis, and fibromyalgia.

The first step in applying functional medicine to clinical practice is recognizing that what appears to be an illness is a state of disharmony resulting from the interplay of antecedents, triggers, and mediators. These concepts have been defined in Chapter 8 of the *Textbook of Functional Medicine*, and we will briefly discuss them here.

Antecedents are any factors, genetic or acquired, that predispose to illness (from the perspective of prevention, they are risk factors). Understanding the antecedents of illness helps the healthcare practitioner understand the unique characteristics of each patient as they relate to his or her current health status. A precipitating event is a critical antecedent that closely precedes the development of chronic illness. It represents a boundary in time: before this event, the person was considered healthy; since the event, the person has become a patient.

A salient characteristic of antecedents and precipitating events is that they *precede* the development of clinical disease but are essential to its formation. Here are 3 examples:

- The genetic predisposition to celiac disease is a critical antecedent to the development of gluten enteropathy and its multiple systemic effects.
- Alterations in the gastrointestinal flora, with a decrease in *Lactobacillus* and *Bifidobacterium* and an increase in *Clostridium* and putrefactive *Bacteroides* species, may contribute to the development of colon cancer. This is an acquired antecedent, influenced to a large extent by diet.
- Reactive arthritis is a systemic inflammatory disorder that follows the development of an acute infection, often an enterocolitis. The acute gastrointestinal infection is a precipitating event leading to a chronic illness that persists after the precipitating event is over.

Triggers are entities or events that provoke an illness or the emergence or exacerbations of symptoms. Common triggers include physical or psychic trauma, microbes, drugs, allergens, foods (or even the act of eating or drinking), environmental toxins, temperature change, stressful life events, adverse social interactions, and powerful memories. For chronic illnesses, multiple interacting triggers are usually present. A salient characteristic of triggers is that their *continued presence* is required for illness exacerbation. Helping patients identify and remove or silence triggers is a key task of the functional medicine practitioner.

The gastrointestinal tract, with its load of microbes and food components, is an important source of triggers for patients with all types of disease. Understanding the role of gut microbes may be complicated by difficulty in ascertaining whether they act as triggers or precipitating events or both. For example:

- Amebic infection may produce an acute or chronic colitis that resolves with treatment. In such a case, acquisition of the infection is the precipitating event, and the amebic organism itself is the discrete trigger.
- Amebic infection may also provoke an exacerbation of chronic ulcerative colitis; following its treatment, the exacerbation resolves and the patient returns to his/her usual state of colitis. The amebic infection was one among many other putative triggers for colitis.
- In another case, amebic infection may precede the development of ulcerative colitis, making it an antecedent, but treatment of amebiasis does not cure the patient's colitis. The intestinal boundary between the intestinal contents and the lamina propria, rich in immune active cells, may be disrupted by the infection, providing a permeable boundary. In such a case, amebiasis leaves behind an environment ripe for potential triggers that may result in exacerbation. Triggers such as colonic auto-antigens can maintain disease activity.

Another salient characteristic of triggers is that they do not cause disease in and of themselves; all triggers exert their effects through the activation of host-derived mediators.

Mediators are intermediaries that contribute to the manifestations of disease. Like triggers, they do not, in and of themselves, cause disease. Mediators vary in form and substance; they may be biochemical (like prostanoids and cytokines), ionic (like hydrogen ions), social (like reinforcement for staying ill), psychological (like fear), or cultural (like beliefs about the nature of illness). Common mediators of illness include hormones, neurotransmitters, neuropeptides, free radicals, fear of pain or loss, poor self-esteem, low perceived self-efficacy, learned helplessness, lack of relevant health information, and social isolation. The most striking characteristic of all mediators is their lack of disease specificity. Each mediator can be implicated in many different and apparently unrelated diseases, and every disease involves multiple mediators in its formation. The most productive area in biomedical research over the past 50 years has been the identification and isolation of the biochemical disease mediators; this research has primarily been used to support the development of drugs that block mediator synthesis or activity.

From the perspective of functional medicine and this monograph, there are 4 salient aspects of mediators that are crucial for clinical practice:

- Mediators are not only agents of illness, they are agents of health. They are intrinsic components of regulatory systems that subserve homeostasis. Any therapeutic strategy based solely upon mediator suppression will produce undesirable effects that result from the disruption of regulatory systems.
- All illness involves multiple interlocking, reinforcing mediators, both biochemical and psychosocial.
- The ebb and flow of mediator activation can be strongly influenced by the common components of life, including circadian and ultradian rhythms, physical activity and exercise, thoughts, hormones, and diet.
- Gut-derived mediators may have systemic effects. Patients with inflammatory bowel disease, for example, are at great risk for osteoporosis. Part of this risk is attributable to malabsorption, weight loss, or the effects of glucocorticoid therapy. A large part of the risk, however, is a direct result of inflammation. Gut-derived inflammatory mediators, especially interleukin-1, stimulate osteoclasts (thereby increasing the rate of bone loss) and inhibit osteoblasts (thereby decreasing the rate of new bone formation).

By utilizing this model, practitioners can approach illness from a perspective that is patient centered. Antecedents, triggers, and mediators are dynamic, interacting components of illness formation specific to an individual. Understanding the unique antecedents, triggers, and mediators that underlie illness or dysfunction in each patient permits therapy to be targeted to the needs of the individual. The conventional diagnosis assigned to the patient may be of value in identifying plausible antecedents, triggers, or mediators, but the diagnosis is not adequate by itself for the designing of patient-centered care.

To further illustrate these concepts, in this chapter, we will outline the current knowledge on antecedents, triggers, and mediators of disease in the 4 conditions discussed in Chapter 3: inflammatory bowel disease, irritable bowel syndrome, rheumatoid arthritis, and fibromyalgia.

Inflammatory Bowel Disease

Antecedents

Several antecedents of (or risk factors for) inflammatory bowel disease have been identified. **Positive family history** is the largest independent risk factor[1]; for first-degree relatives of Crohn's disease patients, the lifetime risk of developing inflammatory bowel disease is 5.2% for non-Jews and 7.8% for Jews, and for relatives of ulcerative colitis patients, the risk is 1.6% for non-Jews and 5.2% for Jews.[2] The absence of simple Mendelian inheritance, however, suggests that multiple gene translational products contribute to the risk,[3] and several susceptibility regions on different chromosomes were found by genome-wide scans.[1, 3] Defects in genes affecting the innate immune system, epithelial barrier function, and the adaptive immune system have been implicated in inflammatory bowel disease.[4]

- Mutations in environmental sensors and their signaling pathways (such as nucleotide-binding oligomerization domain receptors like NOD2, also known as CARD15) may affect the function of the innate immune system; NOD2/CARD15 mutations appear to account for 10% to 15% of Crohn's disease patients.[1] The functional consequence of these mutations appears to be a loss of physiological tolerance to commensal bacteria,[5] although it has also been suggested that these mutations are implicated in the increased gastrointestinal permeability seen in patients with Crohn's disease and their relatives.[6, 7]
- Mutations in genes coding for transporters such as organic cationic transporter (OCT)1 and OCT2[8] may affect gut permeability.[4]
- Mutations in genes involved in adaptive immunity, such as HLA and TNF-α genes,[9, 10] as well as genes encoding for cytokines and cytokine receptors (such as the IL23R gene[11]), may cause an imbalance between regulatory and effector cell immune responses.[4]

Gastrointestinal infection is another well-described antecedent of inflammatory bowel disease. Patients presenting with their first episode of inflammatory bowel disease have often traveled abroad, had an episode of gastrointestinal infection, or taken antibiotics.[12] In a study of risk factors for development of inflammatory bowel disease, twins with either ulcerative colitis or Crohn's disease reported prior recurrent gastrointestinal infections more often than their healthy co-twins; hospitalizations for gastrointestinal infection were also more common, and age at onset of disease was earlier in those who had reported gastrointestinal infection than those who did not.[13]

Because dietary antigens are, next to microbial antigens, the most common luminal antigens, it is not surprising that **dietary factors** may be important disease antecedents. No consensus has emerged, however, regarding the role of dietary patterns as antecedents of inflammatory bowel disease.[1, 14, 15] Though interpreting studies of dietary factors is difficult (most are small and retrospective, involve long-term dietary recall, and often investigate post-illness diets[16]), there is at least suggestive evidence of the following:

- Increased refined sugar intake and high overall carbohydrate intake may precede the development of Crohn's disease.[17, 18]
- Increased consumption of chemically modified fats (such as those found in margarine) may be involved in the etiology of ulcerative colitis.[19]
- High consumption of fast food (typically high in fat that may have been chemically modified) is an antecedent of both ulcerative colitis and Crohn's disease.[20]

- Inert, inorganic, nonnutritive microparticles such as food additives and caking agents—features of the modern urban diet—may combine with gastrointestinal luminal components such as bacterial wall lipopolysaccharides to become antigenic and either initiate disease or trigger disease exacerbations.[21]
- A recent study demonstrated an inverse association between dietary intake of vegetables, fruits, fish, fiber, and omega-3 fatty acids and the subsequent development of Crohn's disease in children.[22]

Formula feeding (or, more specifically, short duration of breast-feeding or the absence of breast-feeding) may be an antecedent of inflammatory bowel disease. Breast-feeding may protect against enteric infections during infancy, aid with early development of a competent gastrointestinal immune system, or delay exposure to foreign antigens such as cow's milk. Several studies have found that people who develop inflammatory bowel disease are less likely to have been breast-fed than controls.[16, 23] **Intolerance to cow's milk** has also been implicated as an antecedent of disease, although the data are somewhat conflicting.[16, 24] In one study, patients with a history of milk allergy during infancy who subsequently developed ulcerative colitis did so at an earlier age than those without a history of milk allergy,[24] and at least one reviewer suggests that "allergy to milk proteins still remains a possible cause of dairy sensitivity or milk intolerance in a small percentage of [inflammatory bowel disease] patients."[16]

Several studies have demonstrated an association between **allergic symptoms, asthma, rhinitis**, and the subsequent development of inflammatory bowel disease, particularly ulcerative colitis.[25-27] The connection between these diseases may relate to the hygiene hypothesis (discussed in Chapter 2).

Abnormal gut permeability is a feature of established inflammatory bowel disease,[6, 28] but there is evidence to suggest that this abnormality precedes the development of frank disease. Studies have demonstrated that relatives of patients with inflammatory bowel disease demonstrate increased permeability (possibly, as discussed above, genetically influenced), suggesting that increased permeability is an antecedent of disease.[6, 28] Although there are very few studies following relatives to assess for subsequent development of inflammatory bowel disease, Irvine and Marshall showed that, in a woman tested because of a family history of Crohn's disease, hyperpermeability preceded the development of frank disease.[29]

Deficiency of vitamin D, a vitamin now widely recognized as a regulator of the immune system, may also be an antecedent of inflammatory bowel disease.[30] The incidence of inflammatory bowel disease is higher at northern latitudes, and both symptomatic onset and relapses occur more commonly in autumn and winter months, when levels of sunlight are low.[30] Further evidence that hypovitaminosis D may be an antecedent comes from animal studies showing that the active form of vitamin D inhibits the development of inflammatory bowel disease and that the absence of the vitamin D receptor is associated with activation of the innate immune system and the development of colitis.[31]

Other factors thought to be antecedents of inflammatory bowel disease include the use of oral contraceptives or hormone replacement therapy,[32, 33] perinatal passive smoke exposure,[34] childhood smoke exposure (passive or active),[35] smoking (for Crohn's disease),[36] prematurity (but not mode of delivery),[37] appendectomy (for Crohn's disease),[38] and treatment of acne with isotretinoin.[39, 40]

Triggers

Infectious agents are well-described triggers of inflammatory bowel disease exacerbations. Indeed, in one study, enteric infections were responsible for 10% of disease flares.[41]

- *Clostridium difficile* is associated with exacerbations, particularly in patients with ulcerative colitis (Crohn's disease patients are more likely to have been treated with metronidazole, which may eradicate *C. difficile*). The incidence of *C. difficile* infection in inflammatory bowel disease patients has increased in recent years; most of the infections are acquired outside the hospital, and many of them are not acquired secondary to antibiotic treatment. *C. difficile* infection negatively impacts clinical outcome in inflammatory bowel disease patients because the associated diarrhea is often thought to represent a noninfectious disease flare and is thus not appropriately treated.[42, 43]

- *Mycobacterium avium* subspecies *paratuberculosis* has also been found in Crohn's disease patients and may be responsible for triggering disease flares. In some patients, it may set the stage for the exacerbation (in this case, it would be an antecedent and then a trigger). *Paratuberculosis* was cultured from the blood of patients with Crohn's disease,[44] and *paratuberculosis* DNA was found in tissue samples[45, 46]; its presence in both inflamed and normal tissue led the authors of one study to speculate that the infection may be systemic, thereby serving as an antecedent.[45] In another study, antibodies against *paratuberculosis* were found in Crohn's disease patients, and the antibody titers correlated with the presence of penetrating or stricture-type disease.[47] Recently it has been suggested that cross-reactivity between *paratuberculosis* and human intestinal proteins may explain the association between mycobacterial infection and Crohn's disease.[48]
- Certain strains of *Escherichia coli* may also trigger disease flares or serve as a disruptor of the system antecedent to the flare. Invasive adherent strains of *E. coli* were found in gut tissue from patients with inflammatory bowel disease, in particular patients with Crohn's disease.[49-52] In one study, the isolated *E. coli* strains were shown *in vitro* to be associated with proinflammatory cytokine expression and decreases in epithelial barrier function.[50] And in a study of *E. coli* in an animal model of inflammatory ileitis, the bacteria induced toll-like receptor sensing and subsequent activation of the innate immune system.[53]
- *Cytomegalovirus* has been found in both blood and intestinal tissue of patients with inflammatory bowel disease[54] and has been detected frequently in patients experiencing acute exacerbations of colitis,[55] thus acting as a trigger.
- *Yersinia enterocolitica* has also been associated with the development of inflammatory bowel disease,[56]acting as both an antecedent and trigger.
- It has recently been hypothesized that infection with a pathogenic variant of *Blastocystis*, which may have been transmitted from the Middle East following its emergence there in the 1980s, may trigger the development of inflammatory bowel disease.[57]
- Other infectious agents that have been found in association with disease exacerbations include *Campylobacter, Entamoeba histolytica, Salmonella, Plesiomonas shigelloides*, and *Strongyloides stercoralis*.[41]

Small bowel bacterial overgrowth may also be a trigger of flares in Crohn's disease.[58, 59] In a study of Crohn's disease patients, up to 20% of patients (and up to 30% of patients with previous surgeries) were found to have small bowel bacterial overgrowth; treatment of the overgrowth resulted in an improvement in bloating, stool consistency, and pain.[60]

It is likely that certain **antigens in food** are responsible for triggering disease exacerbations in at least a subset of Crohn's disease patients. Yeast antigens are widespread components of food and have been implicated in such exacerbations. Antibodies against *Saccharomyces cerevisiae* were found in up to 70% of patients with Crohn's disease, suggesting a loss of tolerance to this dietary antigen.[61, 62] The presence of antibodies is associated with more severe disease, and higher titers have been associated with more rapid development of complications.[61] The exact antigen responsible for the development of these antibodies is unknown, but a recent study suggests *Candida albicans* as a candidate.[63] In a small study, rectal exposure to yeast and citrus antigens produced increased rectal blood flow and submucosal edema in Crohn's disease patients compared to controls.[64]

Clinical Pearl:

Always ask your patients with chronic illness whether they have taken antibiotics for any reason during the course of their illness and how these medications have affected their symptoms. A reduction in symptoms associated with antibiotic use may indicate the presence of bacterial triggers.

In ulcerative colitis, the role of food as a trigger is uncertain. In one study, high intake of meat (particularly red meat and processed meat) and protein was associated with an increased risk of exacerbation in ulcerative colitis patients; high sulfur and sulfate intake was also associated with relapse, and the authors postulated that the sulfur content of high-protein foods and processed foods may influence their ability to trigger exacerbations.[65] In a study in which patients avoided specific foods that they believed triggered symptoms, higher rates of remission were seen at 2 years than in controls.[66] An observational study, however, failed to show an association between patients' avoidance of foods and the risk of relapse.[67]

Nonsteroidal anti-inflammatory drugs (NSAIDs) have been associated with exacerbations of inflammatory bowel disease (both ulcerative colitis and Crohn's disease) in several studies,[68-71] although this is not the case in all studies.[72, 73] Attempts to discover whether the selective COX-2 inhibitors are less likely to cause exacerbations[73, 74] are less relevant in light of the withdrawal of some of these agents from the market. Although relapses are not uniformly associated with NSAID use, there is enough evidence for one reviewer to suggest that NSAIDs "may precipitate a relapse in some patients with inflammatory bowel disease"[75] and for another to suggest that in patients with inflammatory bowel disease, NSAIDs "should be avoided, when possible."[76]

Stress has long been known to be associated with relapses of inflammatory bowel disease,[77-79] although study of this trigger is difficult since it requires teasing out the exact contribution of stressful events, the baseline personality, patient perceptions of events as stressful, and other coincident factors affecting disease activity.[78] Stresses that appear to influence the disease course include those associated with the disease itself, chronic daily life stresses, and acutely stressful events. Depression (which was found to occur at rates triple that of the general population in 2 recent large surveys of patients with inflammatory bowel disease[80]) was noted to exert a negative influence on the course of inflammatory bowel disease and should be considered a predisposing factor for disease relapse.[81]

Mediators

T cells are important mediators in inflammatory bowel disease, but Crohn's disease and ulcerative colitis appear to have different **immune pathways and inflammatory mediators**.[3, 82] In Crohn's disease, the mucosa is dominated by CD4+ lymphocytes with a T-helper-1 (Th1) phenotype; the differentiation into Th1 cells is mediated through interleukin-23.[1] These activated T cells produce and release proinflammatory cytokines such as interleukin-2, -12, and -18 and IFN-γ, which stimulate macrophages to release interleukin-1, interleukin-6, and TNF-α.[1, 3, 82] In contrast, in ulcerative colitis, the mucosa is dominated by atypical T-helper-2 (Th2) cells, characterized by the production of transforming growth factor-beta (TGF-β), as well as interleukin-5 and interleukin-13 and possibly interleukin-4 and interleukin-8.[3, 82, 83]

Mediators of inflammation also may include:

- Leukotriene B4, a potent neutrophil attractor[84]
- Interleukin-6, which facilitates resistance of T cells to apoptosis[85]
- Th17 cells (T-helper cells that produce interleukin-17), which are produced in response to TGF-β[1]
- Antigen-presenting cells, which normally induce anergy in CD4+ T cells; in inflammatory bowel disease, they acquire an activated phenotype in the presence of proinflammatory cytokines such as IFN-γ and TNF-α[1]
- Substance P, which is secreted by macrophages, eosinophils, lymphocytes, and dendritic cells[86]
- Insulin-like growth factors[87]

Activation of these immune cell populations is eventually accompanied by the production of a wide variety of nonspecific mediators of inflammation, including growth factors, prostaglandins, leukotrienes, and reactive oxygen species such as nitric oxide; these mediators all act to enhance inflammation and tissue destruction.[3]

In addition to these mediators of inflammation in the gastrointestinal tract, there are several secondary mediators of morbidity in inflammatory bowel disease patients, including nutritional deficiencies, systemic effects of inflammation, iatrogenic factors, and psychosocial factors.

Nutritional deficiencies are common in inflammatory bowel disease patients and may be due to inadequate dietary intake, malabsorption, or chronic disease activity. In a recent study, patients with inflammatory bowel disease were found to have deficiencies in levels of vitamin E (63%), vitamin D (36%), vitamin A (26%), calcium (23%), folate (19%), iron (13%), vitamin C (11%), hemoglobin (40%), ferritin (39.2%), vitamin B6 (29%), carotene (23.4%), vitamin B12 (18.4%), vitamin D (17.6%), albumin (17.6%), and zinc (15.2%).[88] The authors noted that these deficiencies may be present even in patients who appear well nourished. In another study, serum concentrations of several nutrients (beta-carotene, magnesium, selenium, and zinc) were significantly lower in ulcerative colitis patients compared with controls, and serum vitamin B12 concentrations were significantly lower in Crohn's disease patients.[89]

Key consequences of these nutritional deficiencies include:

- A lack of certain vitamins, notably B12 and folate, are associated with hyperhomocysteinemia. Homocysteine is believed to promote inflammatory processes through its effects on oxidative stress, endoplasmic reticulum stress, and host-microbial interactions, and levels of homocysteine were shown to correlate with disease activity in ulcerative colitis.[90]
- Zinc deficiencies may also be particularly significant. Zinc was shown to regulate gut permeability in animal models of colitis,[91] and zinc supplementation was shown to decrease permeability in patients with quiescent Crohn's disease.[92]
- Magnesium deficiency may lead to cramps, bone pain, fatigue, depression, delirium, and urolithiasis.[93, 94]
- Anemia (which, according to a recent review,[95] occurs in anywhere between 8.8% and 73.7% of patients with inflammatory bowel disease) decreases patient well-being and overall quality of life and is associated with increased hospitalizations.[95] In inflammatory bowel disease, anemia has several causes, including bone marrow suppression and deficiencies of vitamins and iron. Iron deficiency anemia occurs in up one-third of patients[96] and clearly negatively impacts quality of life.

Systemic effects of inflammation that mediate morbidity include oxidative stress, osteoporosis, muscle wasting, hypogonadism, and depression. Reactive oxygen species are produced in abnormally high quantities in patients with inflammatory bowel disease, and it is suggested that they act to mediate (or even possibly trigger) gut inflammation. Reactive oxygen species can increase gut permeability and damage colonic epithelium, thus contributing to the disease process.[97]

Osteoporosis occurs in up to 30% of patients with inflammatory bowel disease[98]; causative factors include malnutrition, immobilization, and steroid use.[98-100] Osteoporosis may predispose to the development of fractures, and the prevalence of vertebral fractures in patients with severely reduced bone density can be up to 22%.[101] The gastrointestinal inflammatory process itself also contributes to bone loss; proinflammatory cytokines produced in inflammatory bowel disease, such as interleukin-1 and TNF-α, displace the balance of bone formation and resorption toward resorption.[98]

Muscle wasting is also a feature of inflammatory bowel disease[102, 103] and clearly contributes to morbidity. Muscle wasting appears to be a systemic effect of gut inflammation, mediated by oxidative stress that is transmitted to remote organs (in this case, muscle) via proinflammatory cytokines such as interleukin-1, interleukin-6, TNF-α, and IFN-γ.[104] Cytokines activate peripheral leucocytes that invade tissue and produce excess oxidants; the oxidants, in turn, may directly damage muscle tissue or may turn on catabolic signals such as reactive oxygen species.[104] Proinflammatory cytokines also were shown to suppress the expression and function of the local anabolic growth factor insulin-like growth factor-1.[105] In addition, the immobility that may be a feature of inflammatory bowel disease can also act on muscle to induce atrophy; atrophy due to immobility or inactivity is strongly linked to oxidative stress.[104]

Hypogonadism is another systemic effect of inflammation seen in several chronic diseases. It can be associated with decreased energy, decreased concentration, decreased memory, depression, and a loss of well-being, as well as the obvious decrease in sexual function; it can also lead to loss of muscle and bone.[106] Hypogonadism that occurs secondary to inflammation may be mediated through TNF-α, interleukin-1, and interleukin-6, which act directly to suppress testicular function and possibly also suppress the hypothalamic-pituitary-gonadal (HPG) axis.[106]

Depression, as noted above, is a common feature of inflammatory bowel disease.[80] While depression may be a psychological response to the presence of chronic disease (and may indeed induce disease exacerbation), there is increasing evidence to suggest that inflammatory processes mediate depression; thus, the inflammatory processes in inflammatory bowel disease may be at least in part responsible for the associated depression. The relationship between immune, autonomic, neuroendocrine, and central neurotransmitter processes is multidirectional.[107] So just as psychological factors may affect immunity, inflammatory mediators (in particular interleukin-1, interleukin-6, and TNF-α) may affect neuroendocrine and neurotransmitter processes, influencing the susceptibility to affective disorders.[107]

In addition to these systemic effects of inflammation, certain **iatrogenic factors** also mediate morbidity in inflammatory bowel disease. Folic acid deficiency is associated with the use of the 5-aminosalicylic acid-based compound sulfasalazine, which interferes with folate transport and is a commonly used treatment[108] (although we must add a note of caution about folate supplementation following the recent report suggesting that it may be associated with carcinogenesis[109]). Methotrexate, another common treatment, is also a folate antagonist.[110] Side effects of other drugs used in the treatment of inflammatory bowel disease are discussed in Chapter 3. For example, corticosteroids have several well-documented side effects, including metabolic, dermatologic, ocular, neuropsychiatric, and immunologic disturbances.[111]

Psychosocial factors also mediate morbidity in inflammatory bowel disease. Patients were shown to have lower quality of life, as well as a lower sense of well-being and mastery, decreased social support, and increased levels of distress and anxiety about their health.[112] The depression that so frequently accompanies the disease was shown to negatively affect response to treatment.[113] Personality traits such as poor tolerance of frustration and perfectionistic body ideal also were shown to negatively affect psychosocial adjustment after surgery.[114] Social and emotional aspects of the quality of life in inflammatory bowel disease patients are influenced by the level of social support received.[115] Unemployment and sick leave are more common in inflammatory bowel disease patients and impact negatively on quality of life.[116]

Irritable Bowel Syndrome

Antecedents

Several studies provide evidence of **familial aggregation** of irritable bowel syndrome, as well as other functional gastrointestinal disorders[117-120]; having a relative with a functional gastrointestinal disorder can thus be considered an antecedent. The relative contribution of genetic predisposition, heightened familial awareness of gastrointestinal symptoms, and shared environmental precipitants is unknown. Research in twins by Levy et al has led to the suggestion that there is a genetic component to the disorder[121]; candidate genes that may be involved include the serotonin transporter gene and the gene that codes for G proteins (an intracellular second messenger signaling protein linked to more than 80% of all membrane receptors).[122, 123] The strongest evidence to date points to a link between serotonin transporter gene polymorphisms and irritable bowel syndrome.[124]

Gastrointestinal infection is a common antecedent of irritable bowel syndrome, and acute bacterial gastroenteritis is the strongest risk factor identified to date for the development of post-infectious irritable bowel syndrome.[125] Up to17% of patients with irritable bowel syndrome believe that their symptoms began with an infection, and prospective studies have shown a 4% to 31% incidence of post-infectious irritable bowel syndrome following an episode of gastroenteritis.[126] A recent study reported that the risk of developing irritable bowel syndrome was twice as high after an acute episode of bacterial gastroenteritis.[127] Female gender, duration of the infectious illness, infection with certain pathogens such as *Shigella* and *Campylobacter*, and poor psychological status all appear to be strong predictors of the development of post-infectious irritable bowel syndrome[128]; smoking may also increase the risk.[129]

Treatment with antibiotics, known to disrupt the composition of the gastrointestinal flora, may be an antecedent of irritable bowel syndrome. Reports of increased development of functional bowel symptoms in patients who had previously received antibiotics for non-gastrointestinal reasons, as well as a recent animal study in which antibiotics induced visceral hypersensitivity, support the contention that antibiotic treatment induces changes in gut flora that predispose to the development of irritable bowel syndrome.[130-132] Since presumably most, if not all, patients diagnosed with bacterial gastroenteritis receive antibiotics, the relative contribution of the infectious agent itself and of treatment with antibiotics to the subsequent development of the disorder cannot be unraveled. In one study, the percentage of people with gastroenteritis treated with antibiotics was similar in both the group that went on to develop irritable bowel syndrome and the group that did not.[133]

Several studies have documented the comorbidity of **asthma** (as well as **allergic rhinitis** in a recent large study) with irritable bowel syndrome.[134-136] In at least one of these studies, the asthma predated the gastrointestinal diagnosis,[135] suggesting that asthma (or atopy) may be an antecedent of irritable bowel syndrome. Other comorbid conditions are very common in patients with irritable bowel syndrome; these conditions include fibromyalgia, chronic fatigue syndrome, temporomandibular joint disorder, chronic pelvic pain, migraine, vulvodynia (chronic vulvar pain), and depression.[137-141] It is within this context of comorbid conditions that a higher incidence of irritable bowel syndrome occurs, suggesting a preceding susceptible biological terrain.

Traumatic experiences in childhood are known antecedents of irritable bowel syndrome. Experiences such as neglect, abuse, loss of a parent, or sexual victimization were shown to be associated with the development of irritable bowel syndrome (as well as depression) later in life.[142-144]

Clinical Pearl:

Try to understand what your patient's health and life were like before the onset of the present illness. Sir William Osler's adage has never been more appropriate: "It is much more important to know what sort of a patient has a disease than what sort of a disease a patient has."

Although dietary factors are known to trigger symptoms in irritable bowel syndrome (see below), there is little evidence to suggest that particular dietary patterns predispose to the development of the condition. Dietary fiber intake has been found in different studies to be similar in irritable bowel syndrome patients and controls,[145] to be similar in total but with a higher intake of simple carbohydrates in patients with irritable bowel syndrome,[146] and to be lower in patients with irritable bowel syndrome.[147] Since many irritable bowel syndrome patients voluntarily restrict their diets in an attempt to ease symptoms, assessing whether dietary patterns predispose to the development of illness or represent responses to symptoms is extremely difficult.

Triggers

Among the most common triggers of irritable bowel syndrome is **food**. In one study, 70% of patients described symptoms related to the intake of food[148]; in another, 62% of patients with irritable bowel syndrome limited or excluded food items from their diet because they were perceived as aggravating symptoms.[148] Indeed, from the patient's perspective, the most frequently perceived cause of symptoms is food; about 50% of patients reported that symptoms are worse after eating, and fully 60% of patients perceive that they have a food allergy and wish to discuss this with their practitioner.[149] A recent study examining food intolerances found an increased rate of positive skin-prick tests to food allergens in irritable bowel syndrome patients.[150] And although antibody and skin-prick tests are not always reliable indicators of which foods are triggering symptoms, in at least one study, elimination of foods based on antibody patterns was associated with an improvement in symptoms.[151]

Infectious agents are also triggers of exacerbations in patients with irritable bowel syndrome. Protozoan infections are associated with irritable bowel syndrome, and they may be antecedents or may trigger symptoms. In one study, *Giardia lamblia* was found in 6.7% of patients presenting with irritable bowel syndrome or functional dyspepsia.[152] Recently, there has been renewed interest in the role of protozoa in irritable bowel syndrome with the discovery that in addition to *Giardia lamblia*, other protozoa such as *B. hominis* and *Dientamoeba fragilis* (both difficult to detect) may be antecedents and triggers of the illness.[153]

Yeasts, and specifically *C. albicans*, may also trigger symptoms in patients with irritable bowel syndrome.[154] Since *Candida* is a normal resident of the gastrointestinal tract, identifying which patients it is responsible for symptoms in is difficult. *Candida* is poly-antigenic, with cross-reactivity to several yeasts and molds; it contains glycoproteins that have the potential to stimulate mast cells to release proinflammatory substances such as histamine and prostaglandin E2; and it can produce proteases that degrade secretory IgA, which is an essential part of the defense provided by gut mucus membranes. These features lend support to the theory that *Candida* may trigger symptoms.[154]

Small bowel bacterial overgrowth has been found in conjunction with irritable bowel syndrome in several studies[155-158] (in 78% of irritable bowel syndrome patients in one study[159]) and may be responsible for several of the symptoms experienced by patients, such as bloating, diarrhea, and abdominal pain. Pimentel et al showed that eradication of the overgrowth resulted in symptom improvement.[156]

Other more subtle **disturbances of gut flora**, including decreases in concentrations of beneficial flora such as *Lactobacillus* and *Bifidobacterium*, have been described in patients with irritable bowel syndrome.[160-162] Administration of probiotics resulted in symptomatic relief in several studies, leading to the suggestion that depletion of beneficial gut flora may be responsible for triggering symptoms.[163-165] Some authors proposed that proliferation of species that produce more gas through fermentation may be responsible for symptoms.[166] The fact that antibiotics change the composition of gut flora also provides additional evidence that antibiotics are a trigger of irritable bowel syndrome.

Stressful life events are well-recognized symptom triggers in patients with irritable bowel syndrome, and stress has been shown, in both animal and human studies, to affect gastrointestinal motility and sensitivity in this disorder.[167] In one study, chronic stress (longer than 6 months' duration) related to events like divorce or other relationship problems, illness, business failures, job losses, and lawsuits correlated strongly with subsequent symptoms; no patient who had experienced even one of these chronic stressors improved clinically over the subsequent study period (16 months).[168] It is not only extreme stress, however, that triggers symptoms; more minor, everyday stresses also were found to correlate with an increase in symptoms.[169] Not surprisingly, symptoms can also aggravate stress levels.[170]

Mediators

Irritable bowel syndrome involves **inflammatory cascades**, the **enteric nervous system**, the **autonomic nervous system**, and the **central nervous system**, and the list of putative mediators is long and complex.

- The neurotransmitter serotonin appears to play a central role. Ninety-five percent of the body's serotonin is located in the gastrointestinal tract (within enterochromaffin cells, neurons, mast cells, and smooth muscle cells),[171] and serotonin is intimately involved in the signaling between enterochromaffin cells and sensory nerve fibers in the mucosal layer of the gut.[172] Upon release by enterochromaffin cells, serotonin stimulates extrinsic vagal afferent nerve fibers and intrinsic enteric afferent nerve fibers, causing physiological responses such as intestinal secretion, peristalsis, and bloating.[171]
- Mediators secreted by mast cells have also been implicated in the production of stress-induced symptoms in irritable bowel syndrome (hypothesized by one author to occur through the effect of stress on gut barrier function, which increases access of sensitizing agents to enteric mast cells).[173] Marked increases in numbers of mast cells were found in the jejunal mucosa of patients with diarrhea-predominant irritable bowel syndrome, who had higher levels of stress than controls.[174] In the presence of sensitizing antigens, mast cells can release a broad mix of preformed chemical mediators including histamine, interleukin-6, leukotrienes, platelet activating factor, proteoglycans, and prostaglandins, all of which can act on receptors in the enteric

nervous system and activate "silent" sensory nerves.[174] A recent animal study demonstrated that mediators released from mast cells in tissue taken from irritable bowel syndrome patients resulted in increased firing of visceral-nociceptive sensory neurons in rats.[175]

- Other neurotransmitters that may be involved include vasoactive intestinal polypeptide,[176] acetylcholine, nitric oxide, substance P, and pituitary adenylate cyclase-activating polypeptide.[171]
- A 2005 animal study of post-infectious irritable bowel syndrome found the continued presence of TGF-β1 in jejunal muscle, with subsequent upregulation of COX-2 and prostaglandin E2, suggesting that these substances mediate the hypercontractility seen in irritable bowel syndrome.[177]
- The hypothalamic-pituitary-adrenal (HPA) axis provides a link between the brain and the gut immune system and thus may be implicated as a mediator. Increased concentrations of cortisol and the proinflammatory cytokines interleukin-6 and interleukin-8 were found in patients with irritable bowel syndrome, along with increased levels of adrenocorticotropic hormone (ACTH) and cortisol following corticotrophin-releasing hormone infusion. It has been suggested that overactivity of the HPA axis, associated with increases in interleukin-6 and -8, mediates disorder in irritable bowel syndrome.[178]

In addition to these mediators, there are secondary mediators of morbidity in patients with irritable bowel syndrome. **Food intolerance** is a central feature of irritable bowel syndrome, and patients often limit or exclude certain foods from their diet; **nutritional deficiencies** from diarrhea or voluntary dietary restriction, therefore, can occur. In one study, patients excluded a wide variety of foods from their diet, including dairy products (particularly milk), vegetables, fruits, nuts, cereals, and meat.[148] Not surprisingly, 12% of patients were deemed to have an "inadequate diet."[148]

Psychosocial factors are also clearly important mediators of morbidity, particularly in the case of an illness such as irritable bowel syndrome which, despite great advances in medical knowledge regarding pathophysiology in recent years, is still considered by many to be not a "real" disease. Negative sociocultural perception of the disorder may negatively affect patients' perception of themselves, their symptoms, and their illness. Interaction among biological, psychological, and social factors determines each patient's experience of the illness.[179] For instance, the perceived severity of irritable bowel syndrome symptoms depends on several factors, including who makes the assessment (patient or physician) and how much impairment or disability is associated with the symptoms. Perceived severity can markedly affect health-related quality of life, healthcare utilization behaviors, and burden of illness.[180]

Stressful responses to symptoms, inability to go about daily life, and fear about such things as the risk of developing cancer are common among patients with irritable bowel syndrome and increase feelings of illness and healthcare-seeking behavior.[181] "Catastrophizing," or magnification of pain-related stimuli in association with feelings of helplessness and pessimism, increases depression, as well as severity of pain.[182] Feelings of control (or lack of control) over the disorder are also important. An 8-session self-management program for women with irritable bowel syndrome that taught techniques such as coping strategies, relaxation, abdominal breathing, and problem-solving skills was effective in reducing symptoms, as well as improving quality of life and reducing psychological distress[183]; even a single session of reassurance can improve perceptions of impairment.[181]

Rheumatoid Arthritis

Antecedents

A **family history** of rheumatoid arthritis is an antecedent of disease, although the contribution of genetic factors appears to be modest.[184] The most important genetic factor found to date is within the HLA system, yet non-HLA genes have also been implicated.[184, 185] Several HLA-DRB1 alleles are associated with disease predisposition.[185] Non-HLA genes thought to be important include those for corticotrophin-releasing hormone, estrogen synthase, IFN-γ, and a variety of cytokines.[184]

There has long been intense interest in the possible role of **infectious agents** in the pathogenesis of rheumatoid arthritis, and several infectious agents have been proposed as disease antecedents.

- *Mycoplasma* infection may be a disease antecedent; *Mycoplasma* species were detected in the blood of patients with rheumatoid arthritis,[184] and *Mycoplasma* antibodies were detected in both blood[186, 187] and synovial fluid.[188, 189] *Mycoplasma* also was shown to induce experimental arthritis in rabbits.[190]
- There is evidence to suggest that infection with *Proteus mirabilis*, possibly originating in the urinary tract, is an antecedent.[191, 192]
- Other authors feel that the evidence points more toward Epstein-Barr virus as a disease antecedent. In one study, the DNA load of Epstein-Barr virus was 10 times higher in the peripheral blood mononuclear cells of rheumatoid arthritis patients than controls, and the virus also was detected in synovial fluid.[193]
- In a case report, *Chlamydia trachomatis* monoarticular infection in a young woman preceded a diagnosis of rheumatoid arthritis.[194]
- *E. histolytica* has also been suggested as a disease antecedent,[195] and DNA from a variety of other bacterial species (including *Neisseria, Acinetobacter, Moraxella, Salmonella,* and *Pseudomonas*) has been isolated from the synovial fluid of rheumatoid arthritis patients, although the significance is unclear.[196]

One author postulated that any one of a number of "arthritogenic" intestinal bacteria may be, for genetic reasons, more common in patients who eventually develop rheumatoid arthritis; continual seeding of bacterial products from the gut leads to synovial inflammation, erosion of joint surfaces, exposure of cartilage antigens, and autoimmunity.[197]

Abnormalities in both the HPA axis and the HPG axis have been found in patients with rheumatoid arthritis,[198, 199] and these abnormalities may be antecedents of disease. Both adrenal and gonadal hormones are known to affect the cells involved in inflammatory responses, and inflammatory cytokines such as interleukin-1 and interleukin-6 also modulate the function of the HPA axis and the HPG axis; interactions among all these systems mediate the response to stressors.[198] Intact ACTH secretion with impaired adrenal response to ACTH characterizes rheumatoid arthritis; the overall activity of the HPA axis was described as "inappropriately normal" in these patients and insufficient to inhibit inflammation. The decreased cortisol levels are present despite high levels of interleukin-6, which should stimulate cortisol release.[200] In particular, young women who have been affected by ongoing stressful events (such as interpersonal stress, surgery, infection) and who have low adrenal responsiveness to these stressors are candidates for subsequent development of rheumatoid arthritis.[198] Decreased levels of adrenal androgens also were found, further supporting the role of relative adrenal insufficiency as a disease antecedent.[198]

Decreased levels of gonadal androgens (which are natural anti-inflammatory substances) have also been found in rheumatoid arthritis, implying abnormalities in the HPG axis and supporting a possible antecedent role for deficiencies of these immunosuppressive androgens.[198] And although serum estrogen levels are normal in patients with rheumatoid arthritis, it is suggested that changes in the sex hormone milieu or in the peripheral conversion of estrogens (such as occurs during the postpartum period) may also be antecedents of rheumatoid arthritis.[193, 198, 201] Women are 10 times more likely to develop rheumatoid arthritis in the postpartum period compared with other time periods,[201] and women are also more likely to develop the disease during the perimenopausal period.[201] Nulliparity also was shown to increase the risk for later development of rheumatoid arthritis.[201]

Knowledge about the role of **dietary factors** as antecedents of rheumatoid arthritis (and other arthritides) continues to evolve and are discussed in a 2005 review.[202] Several studies have suggested a link between the intake of red meat and the risk of development of rheumatoid arthritis,[202] although a recent study failed to find an association.[203] Other studies have suggested that aspects of the Mediterranean diet (high consumption of olive oil, fruit, vegetables, nuts, legumes, whole-grain cereals, and fish) may protect against the development of rheumatoid arthritis and, conversely, that diets low in vegetables and fruits increase the risk.[202] Intake of vitamin D also was found to be inversely related to the risk of developing rheumatoid arthritis[204]; it has been suggested that a low level of vitamin D, secondary to either low dietary intake or low exposure to ultraviolet radiation, is a disease antecedent and that vitamin D may protect against the development of rheumatoid arthritis (as well as other autoimmune diseases).[204-206]

It has been suggested, based on observations about rheumatic joint disease among artists (including Rubens and Renoir), that **heavy metal toxicity** (from high concentrations of mercury, cadmium, arsenic, lead, antimony, tin, cobalt, manganese, and chromium found in some paints) may be an antecedent of rheumatoid arthritis.[207]

Smoking is increasingly being recognized as an antecedent of rheumatoid arthritis, and the risk may also apply to people passively exposed to cigarette smoke. The risk appears to diminish after the cessation of smoking, with a relative risk of 1.5 even up to 19 years after quitting.[193] Smoking appears to interact with HLA-DR shared epitope genes to trigger and perpetuate immunity against citrullinated proteins—in other words, there is a gene-environment interaction with respect to smoking that predisposes to the development of disease.[208]

Triggers

As discussed in Chapter 2, a certain subset of patients with rheumatoid arthritis respond to dietary changes, suggesting a role for **gut permeability** or **dysbiosis**. In fact, older studies suggest that the normal intestinal flora of rheumatoid arthritis patients have arthropathic properties when tested in animal models.[209] In human trials, rheumatoid arthritis patients placed on vegetarian diets had decreased disease activity and improved nutritional status.[210-211] Assessment of fecal flora differed significantly before and after dietary modification[212]; in fact, improvement in disease activity occurred only in those patients for whom the diet altered stool bacterial composition. Additionally, these patients had a significant reduction in the mean anti-*Proteus* antibody titers compared to patients who followed an omnivorous diet.[213] Other studies suggest that these antibody levels are highly statistically significant when rheumatid arthritis patients are compared with healthy controls.[214] (For more information on gut dysregulation in rheumatoid arthritis, see *Disease Manifestations of Dysbiosis, Permeability, and Immune Dysregulation* in Chapter 2.)

Daily life stressors such as workplace stress, interpersonal stress, and financial problems have been found to result in worsening of symptoms (pain, physical disability) and signs of disease activity (tender point counts) in rheumatoid arthritis patients.[199] **Physical stress**, such as physical exercise, also was shown to be associated with increased progression of joint damage (although exercise can also be beneficial).[215] Short bouts of exhaustive physical exercise were shown in patients with rheumatoid arthritis to be associated with abnormal cortisol, prolactin, and CD4+/CD8+ T-cell responses to exercise, which may affect disease activity and progression.[216]

Events that change the hormonal milieu can, as discussed above in the context of disease antecedents, predispose to disease exacerbations in rheumatoid arthritis. Symptoms may worsen during the postpartum period (a period of relative adrenal and gonadal insufficiency).[201]

Mediators

Activation of T cells is believed to be the earliest pathological event in rheumatoid arthritis.[217] The disease is classically considered to be driven by Th1 cells, with the lack of Th2 cytokines leading to induction and maintenance of inflammation.[218] Recently, attention has focused on a new CD4+ T-cell subset known as Th17 cells. Activation of these T cells, in conjunction with defective function of regulatory T cells in the synovial inflammatory milieu, appears to be a central event in the disease process.[218]

Inflammatory mediators of tissue damage include:

- Macrophages secrete several inflammatory mediators, including chemokines, cytokines, growth factors, and proteases, all of which mediate the inflammation, angiogenesis, fibrosis, and bone destruction of rheumatoid arthritis.[219]
- Interleukin-1, interleukin-6, and TNF-α are the major proinflammatory cytokines involved in mediating rheumatoid arthritis.[198, 219] Interleukin-12, -15, and -18, which are involved in Th1 polarization, also have

been implicated. In addition, there appears to be a diminished response of macrophages to interleukin-10; the normal response involves activation of IFN-γ.[219]

- Recent research has uncovered the importance of other "novel" cytokines such as interleukin-17, which drives the differentiation of Th17 cells (discussed above); interleukin-20 and interleukin-22, which have proinflammatory effects on fibroblasts; and interleukin-32.[220]
- Other macrophage- and fibroblast-derived factors that mediate damage include those that induce fibroblast proliferation such as platelet-derived growth factor, vascular endothelial growth factor, and TGF-β.[217]
- Mast cells also have a critical role in the pathogenesis of rheumatoid arthritis.[221] Large numbers of activated (degranulated) mast cells are found in the synovial tissue of rheumatoid arthritis patients. These cells release and produce key mediators of inflammation, in particular TNF-α and leukotriene B4; they also stimulate other cells, including fibroblasts and endothelial cells, that contribute to joint damage.[221]

In addition to these mediators of tissue damage, several secondary mediators play a role in the morbidity associated with rheumatoid arthritis. These include **deficiencies of trace elements** such as zinc and magnesium, cofactors in metabolic processes involving collagen and bone or immune system function.[222] Zinc deficiency was reported (although not consistently) in rheumatoid arthritis patients, and treatment with zinc was shown to improve (although not consistently) parameters such as morning stiffness, patient assessment of disease activity, and swelling.[222] Low plasma levels of magnesium also were found in rheumatoid arthritis,[223] and patients were found to have low dietary intake of both magnesium and zinc.[224]

Anemia is a common finding in rheumatoid arthritis (60% to 70% in some studies).[225, 226] The anemia can be an iron-deficiency type, secondary to gastrointestinal losses caused by NSAIDs or nutritional deficiency, or can be an anemia with adequate iron stores—the "anemia of chronic disease."[225, 226] Data suggest that anemia contributes substantially to decreased quality of life among patients with rheumatoid arthritis. Anemia may also possibly be a factor in disease activity, as some studies have found such correlations, as well as improvements in disease activity upon correction of anemia.[225, 226]

Systemic effects of inflammation also mediate morbidity in rheumatoid arthritis. Reactive oxygen species produced during the course of disease exceed the physiological buffering capacity and result in oxidative stress. Excessive production of reactive oxygen species damages protein, lipids, nucleic acid, and matrix components; reactive oxygen species also act as intracellular signaling molecules that amplify the synovial inflammatory response.[227] The end result is persistence of inflammatory synovitis.

Osteoporosis, occurring both as part of the inflammatory process and as a side effect of steroid treatment, contributes to a dramatic decrease in quality of life in rheumatoid arthritis patients, although it is seldom looked for or treated.[228] It is particularly common in older women and correlates with weakness and physical inactivity. The loss of bone mass can occur early in the disease process and is more severe with uncontrolled disease.[228] Not surprisingly, fractures are also considerably more common in patients with rheumatoid arthritis, especially hip and vertebral fractures; the risk increases with increasing functional impairment.[228]

Nearly two thirds of patients with rheumatoid arthritis experience a muscle wasting condition known as rheumatoid cachexia, which compromises muscle strength and is believed to be an important contributor to morbidity and even mortality in these patients. The exact mechanisms are unknown; TNF-α and interleukin-1β are believed to be the central mediators, although low habitual physical activity and reduced peripheral insulin activity may also contribute.[229]

Depression is common in patients with rheumatoid arthritis, occurring in 41% of patients in one study. [230] It is associated with decreased quality of life, as well as poor outcomes in terms of both disease progression and adaptation to treatment.[230] As discussed above under inflammatory bowel disease, the known association between cytokines and depression[231] and the known interactions among nervous, endocrine, and immune systems make it reasonable to suggest that the depression seen in rheumatoid arthritis may be mediated at least in part by the cytokines responsible for the joint disease.

Iatrogenic mediators of morbidity include folic acid deficiency secondary to the use of methotrexate; as discussed above under inflammatory bowel disease, methotrexate is a folic acid antagonist. Side effects of methotrexate include gastrointestinal intolerance, mouth ulcers, cytopenia, alopecia, liver function abnormalities, bone marrow toxicity, and interstitial pneumonitis; several of these side effects (which are similar to those seen in folate depletion) may be secondary to folate antagonism.[232]

Steroid treatment, as discussed in Chapter 3, may also result in significant morbidity. Side effects are numerous, dose related, and well described; they include increased susceptibility to infection, hypoadrenalism, hypogonadism, atherosclerosis, dermatologic abnormalities, muscle wasting,[229] and osteoporosis[228] (which may occur, along with weight gain and ecchymoses, even at low doses of prednisone[233]).[217]

Clinical Pearl:

Almost half the prescription drugs used in clinical practice deplete specific nutrients, impairing the biological responses that regulate inflammatory mediators. Practitioners should take a careful drug history and maintain up-to-date knowledge of drug-induced nutrient depletion and potential drug-supplement interactions.

Psychosocial factors are also important mediators of morbidity in rheumatoid arthritis. The perception of the illness and ability to cope with disease vary greatly among patients and can have a large impact on adaptation to disease; in fact, perception of illness was found to outweigh the impact of medical treatment on depression, physical function, and pain in rheumatoid arthritis patients.[234] Catastrophizing negatively affects the perception of pain and the experience of disease in patients with rheumatoid arthritis (as well as irritable bowel syndrome, as discussed above).[235] Patients under perceived stress who do not use active coping strategies have greater psychological comorbidity,[236] and patients with a prior history of depressive episodes have more pain both at baseline and in response to stress.[237] Support, or lack of support, also influences adaptation to disease in rheumatoid arthritis; perception of a positive spousal response to disease was shown to increase the ability to deal with pain.[238]

Fibromyalgia

Antecedents

Familial clustering has been demonstrated in fibromyalgia, and having a relative with fibromyalgia can be considered an antecedent.[239-242] Although shared environmental factors and learned responses may be responsible in part for this phenomenon, it is becoming clear that **genetic factors** have a significant role in fibromyalgia.[242] Alterations in the serotonin transporter gene, dopamine receptor genes, the gene for catechol-O-methyltransferase (the principal metabolite of norepinephrine), and the gene for the substance P receptor were all suggested as candidate genes.[242]

Many practitioners find that patients with fibromyalgia feel better when they decrease or eliminate sugar and refined flour, independent of food allergies or other issues, suggesting that a **high-glycemic-index diet** is a potential antecedent. In one study, an increased incidence of fibromyalgia was reported among patients with diabetes (either type 1 or 2), and the severity of the fibromyalgia correlated with lack of glycemic control, suggesting that high blood glucose also may be an antecedent of fibromyalgia.[243]

There have been several reports documenting an association between **atopic disorders** and fibromyalgia. Allergic rhinitis, "allergic background," asthma, and eczema all were found in association with fibromyalgia.[244-246] Since atopic disorders often develop in childhood, these disorders may be antecedents of fibromyalgia.

The similarity in the symptoms of both **viral infections** and fibromyalgia (myalgia, fatigue) has stimulated research into the possible role of infections as antecedents of fibromyalgia.

- There is an association between Lyme disease (an infectious disease caused by *Borrelia burgdorferi*) and the subsequent development of symptoms suggestive of fibromyalgia, and it is generally accepted that Lyme disease may be an antecedent of fibromyalgia[247] (although there is also evidence to suggest that the pattern of symptoms may represent a condition—post-Lyme borreliosis syndrome—separate from fibromyalgia[248]).
- Similarly, a high incidence of infection with *Mycoplasma* species in patients with fibromyalgia and/or chronic fatigue syndrome was demonstrated.[247, 249, 250]
- Infection with hepatitis B and C and with HIV was associated with the development of fibromyalgia.[247, 251]
- *Enterovirus* has been found in the skeletal muscle of fibromyalgia patients, suggesting a role in the pathogenesis of the disorder.[252]

In addition to these specific viruses, it has been suggested that chronic viral infection with other as yet unspecified viruses may precede the development of fibromyalgia; these infectious agents may interact with genetic and environmental factors to produce the spectrum of symptoms known as fibromyalgia.[247]

Although there is scarce information dealing specifically with **parasitic infection** as an antecedent of fibromyalgia, there have been reports of infection with intestinal parasites predisposing to the development of other nonspecific chronic illnesses such as chronic fatigue syndrome, which shares many features with fibromyalgia. In one study, infection with *G. lamblia* was found in 61 of 218 patients presenting with chronic fatigue, myalgia, sweats, and other flulike symptoms (indeed, 61% of the patients subsequently found to have giardiasis had been diagnosed with chronic fatigue immune dysfunction syndrome); cure of giardiasis was associated with complete resolution or some improvement in symptoms in 88% of patients.[253] Similarly, eradication of *B. hominis* was shown to improve symptoms in patients previously diagnosed with chronic fatigue immune dysfunction syndrome.[254] And a cluster of patients with symptoms consistent with chronic fatigue syndrome following an episode of giardiasis in a town in California further suggests that infection with *G. lamblia* can predate chronic fatigue syndrome or other similar illnesses.[255]

Altered functioning of the HPA axis may also be an antecedent of fibromyalgia, although reports on the nature of the disturbance are conflicting. Decreases in ACTH response to a variety of stressors such as hypoglycemia, interleukin-6, or exercise were documented, as well as decreases in peak cortisol responses to ACTH,[256] suggesting that the HPA axis is underactive in patients with fibromyalgia and that some patients have subnormal adrenocortical function, possibly as an adaptation to chronic stress.[256]

Low vitamin D levels have also been found in patients with fibromyalgia, in particular in association with depression and anxiety, suggesting that hypovitaminosis D may be an antecedent.[257, 258]

Both **physical and emotional trauma** and **stressful life events** appear to be antecedents (or triggers) of fibromyalgia.

- Motor vehicle accidents, for example, were found (probably acting as stressors rather than through direct mechanical injury) to trigger the development of fibromyalgia.[259]
- Other past physical traumas recalled by patients with fibromyalgia include surgery, childbirth, falls, fractures, and abuse as a child.[260]
- Female adolescents with posttraumatic stress disorder are more likely to have fibromyalgia (as well as other chronic disorders such as chronic fatigue syndrome, irritable bowel syndrome, and chronic pelvic pain).[261]
- Veterans of the Gulf War have a high incidence of Gulf War syndrome, a symptom constellation that shares many similarities with fibromyalgia. It has been postulated that the combination of the multiple vaccinations given to soldiers before they travelled to the Persian Gulf, in combination with the extreme stress of combat, predispose to the development of this fibromyalgia-like disease.[247]
- An overactive "action-prone" lifestyle may also be an antecedent of fibromyalgia.[262]

There are several disorders that frequently coexist with fibromyalgia, suggesting that these disorders may share common antecedents.

- Chronic fatigue syndrome, irritable bowel syndrome, temporomandibular disorder, tension and migraine headaches (especially in women), interstitial cystitis, multiple chemical sensitivities, chronic pelvic pain, chronic vulvar pain (vulvodynia), and endometriosis are frequently associated with fibromyalgia.[246, 263-265]
- Psychiatric comorbidities include generalized anxiety disorder, hypomanic disorder, and, in particular, major depressive disorder.[266, 267]
- An association between systemic lupus erythematosus and fibromyalgia also was reported, with up to 47% of patients with systemic lupus exhibiting symptoms consistent with fibromyalgia.[268]
- Autoimmune thyroiditis also was found in a high percentage of fibromyalgia patients.[269] It has been suggested that fibromyalgia is caused by a resistance, either genetic or acquired, to thyroid hormone; these authors suggest that coagulopathies, possibly secondary to chronic infection, lead to thyroid hormone resistance.[270]

Triggers

Many fibromyalgia patients feel that certain **foods** exacerbate symptoms. In one survey, 42% of patients reported aggravation after ingestion of certain foods, including meat, alcohol, coffee, sweets, sugar, chocolate, citrus fruits, and apples; 23% of patients had tried diet therapy to alleviate symptoms.[271] Other reported triggers include dietary excitotoxins such as monosodium glutamate and aspartame.[272] It has been proposed that a profound loss of tolerance to a particular chemical or food occurs following either acute or chronic exposure and that further exposure to small quantities of the offending chemical or food triggers symptoms. This has been suggested to explain symptoms such as those seen in fibromyalgia, as well as Gulf War syndrome, chronic fatigue syndrome, depression, and other symptom constellations noted above to be comorbidities of fibromyalgia.[273]

Infectious agents may also trigger symptoms. Pimentel et al found that small intestinal bacterial overgrowth was common in fibromyalgia (and more common than in irritable bowel syndrome); the degree of overgrowth (as measured by hydrogen production) correlated with pain.[274] As discussed above, infection with *G. lamblia* or *B. hominis* may trigger symptoms or precede the disease. Chronic infection with *C. albicans* has also been suggested as a possible trigger of chronic fatigue syndrome.[275] It has also been suggested that chronic candidiasis leads to a condition of immune depression that allows reactivation of previously latent infectious agents.[275]

Viral agents such as Epstein-Barr virus, Ross River virus, dengue virus, Coxsackie virus, *Parvovirus*, hepatitis C, hepatitis B, HIV, and HHV-6[255, 276-278] have all been implicated as triggering the onset of fibromyalgia. It has been suggested that certain ubiquitous viruses (such as Epstein-Barr virus and HPV-6) may be reactivated during outbreaks of chronic fatigue syndrome (and by extension, fibromyalgia).[255] Bacterial agents such as *Chlamydia trachomatis* and *Chlamydia pneumoniae*,[279] *Coxiella burnetii* (Q fever),[276] *Borrelia burgdorferi* (Lyme disease), and *Mycoplasma*[247] were all suggested as triggers. It must be pointed out, however, that the role of infection in fibromyalgia continues to be a source of debate; it is not clear whether fibromyalgia coexists with chronic infection or whether infection triggers fibromyalgia.[247]

Physical activity such as exercise may cause increased pain in fibromyalgia patients.[280-282] This abnormal modulation of the response to exercise may be secondary either to increased pain perception at muscle nociceptive afferent nerves or to abnormalities in descending pain-inhibitory pathways.[282] Temporal summation, or "wind-up" (the phenomenon whereby, after an initial painful stimulus, further stimuli are perceived as more painful), is normally attenuated after exercise; in patients with fibromyalgia, abnormal temporal summation results in increased perception of pain after exercise.[280] In addition, patients who are deconditioned due to their illness may experience more muscle microtrauma during exercise, which can lead to increased generalized pain.[283]

Stressful life events can also trigger exacerbations in patients with fibromyalgia. In one study, 65% of patients reported that stress aggravated symptoms; poor sleep, exercise, and cold also aggravated symptoms.[284]

Mediators

Since fibromyalgia is such a complex disorder, probably involving dysfunction at several interconnected levels including the **HPA axis, central pain pathways**, and **immune systems**, the list of potential mediators is long.

- The sympathetic nervous system is known to be intimately involved with fibromyalgia, particularly in the response to stress.[285] Patients with fibromyalgia demonstrate chronically increased sympathetic activation, with decreased response to stress.[285] It has been suggested that fibromyalgia patients have less effective function of catechol-O-methyltransferase, the enzyme responsible for clearing sympathetic catecholamines via methylation and oxidative deamination; this would result in increased levels of the sympathetic catecholamines norepinephrine, epinephrine, and dopamine.[285]
- It is widely accepted that enhanced excitability of the spinal cord neurons that transmit nociceptive information to the brain is a central feature of fibromyalgia, as well as dysregulation of descending pain inhibitory pathways.[286] Serotonin exerts an inhibitory effect on pain pathways, and low levels of serotonin may mediate increased pain perception, especially in patients with coexistent anxiety.[286, 287] Dysregulation of dopamine release in response to pain also was suggested as a mediator of increased pain perception.[288] Substance P, a neuropeptide that was found in increased quantities in the cerebrospinal fluid of patients with fibromyalgia and the release of which is inhibited by serotonin, may also mediate pain perception.[287, 289]
- Glial cells play a substantial role in the modulation of pain signaling. Activated by neurotransmitters, glial cells express receptors for viruses and bacteria; release neuroactive substances such as nitric oxide, prostaglandins, and leukotrienes in response to painful stimuli; release proinflammatory cytokines such as interleukin-1, interleukin-6, and TNF-α; and upregulate release of substance P and other excitatory amino acids from primary afferent neurons. They may play a role in fibromyalgia, although direct evidence is currently lacking.[286]
- Higher levels of interleukin-10, interleukin-8, and TNF-α were found in the plasma of patients with fibromyalgia; significant correlations were found between these biochemical parameters and clinical manifestations, suggesting that these are mediators.[290] Interleukin-1, interleukin-6, and TNF-α were detected in the skin of fibromyalgia patients, suggesting the presence of inflammatory foci.[291]

In addition to these mediators, several secondary events may mediate morbidity in fibromyalgia. **Nutritional deficiencies** may be a factor; increased concentrations of homocysteine, correlating with decreased levels of vitamin B12, were found in the cerebrospinal fluid of fibromyalgia patients, and the levels of B12 correlated with fatigability, suggesting that low B12 levels contribute to symptomatology in these patients.[292] Magnesium deficits, based on response to magnesium loading, were reported in patients with fibromyalgia (and other conditions characterized by chronic fatigue such as chronic fatigue syndrome and spasmophilia).[293] Since magnesium is intimately involved with immune function and stress responses, magnesium deficiency may mediate morbidity.[294]

Other mediators of morbidity include the **side effects of the many medications** commonly used to treat this disorder. (See Chapter 3, *Conventional Approaches to Treatment of Gastrointestinal and Systemic Diseases*.)

Inappropriate physical therapy can increase morbidity in these patients. Since patients with fibromyalgia are often in poor physical condition because of their illness, prescribing intensive exercise may cause problems. Microtraumatic injury to muscles during vigorous exercise may cause localized pain and may trigger widespread pain through disordered central processing.[283] In addition, the postulated abnormal pain processing (discussed above) may contribute to pain experienced during physical exercise.

Psychosocial factors also mediate morbidity in fibromyalgia. Fear of pain and activity (which was shown to be an excellent predictor of disability) is common among fibromyalgia patients and correlates with depression.[295] Illness-focused coping strategies such as guarding, resting, and asking for assistance also were shown to correlate with disability and decreased quality of life.[296] Catastrophizing may have a negative impact on patients with fibromyalgia, resulting in increased reported pain severity, increased tenderness, increased disability, and poor treatment outcome.[235] Psychological well-being, which was shown to be lower in a study of women with fibromyalgia, correlates negatively with disability and fatigue. Self-acceptance, a sense of mastery over one's environment, a sense of purpose in life, and positive relations with others are important factors in the association between psychological well-being and disability.[297] Symptoms such as disturbances in sleep and mental acuity also were reported to result in withdrawal from paid work and from recreational life activities of women with fibromyalgia.[298]

Summary

In this chapter, we introduced the concepts of antecedents, triggers, and mediators of disease as tools to help practitioners move toward a more individualized approach to patient care. We noted how, for any individual patient, multiple antecedents, triggers, and mediators interact to produce dysfunction. And we elaborated on the antecedents, triggers, and mediators of inflammatory bowel disease, irritable bowel syndrome, rheumatoid arthritis, and fibromyalgia. In the next chapter, we will discuss how to use this knowledge of antecedents, triggers, and mediators in the context of the Functional Medicine Matrix Model in order to move away from a model of disease-centered care and toward a collaborative model of patient-centered care. Using this model, healthcare practitioners can assess these multiple interacting components for each patient and strive to restore function and balance by manipulation of each patient's particular antecedents, triggers, and mediators.

References

1. Baumgart DC, Carding SR. Inflammatory bowel disease: cause and immunobiology. *Lancet.* 2007;369:1627-1640.
2. Russell RK, Satsangi J. IBD: a family affair. *Best Pract Res Clin Gastroenterol.* 2004;18:525-539.
3. Podolsky DK. Inflammatory bowel disease. *N Engl J Med.* 2002;347:417-429.
4. Goyette P, Labbe C, Trinh TT, Xavier RJ, Rioux JD. Molecular pathogenesis of inflammatory bowel disease: genotypes, phenotypes and personalized medicine. *Ann Med.* 2007;39:177-199.
5. Quaglietta L, te Velde A, Staiano A, Troncone R, Hommes DW. Functional consequences of NOD2/CARD15 mutations in Crohn disease. *J Pediatr Gastroenterol Nutr.* 2007;44:529-539.
6. Buhner S, Buning C, Genschel J, et al. Genetic basis for increased intestinal permeability in families with Crohn's disease: role of CARD15 3020insC mutation? *Gut.* 2006;55:342-347.
7. Schreiber S. Slipping the barrier: how variants in CARD15 could alter permeability of the intestinal wall and population health. *Gut.* 2006;55:308-309.
8. Peltekova VD, Wintle RF, Rubin LA, et al. Functional variants of OCTN cation transporter genes are associated with Crohn disease. *Nat Genet.* 2004;36:471-475.
9. Yap LM, Ahmad T, Jewell DP. The contribution of HLA genes to IBD susceptibility and phenotype. *Best Pract Res Clin Gastroenterol.* 2004;18:577-596.
10. Fowler EV, Eri R, Hume G, et al. TNFalpha and IL10 SNPs act together to predict disease behaviour in Crohn's disease. *J Med Genet.* 2005;42:523-528.
11. Duerr RH, Taylor KD, Brant SR, et al. A genome-wide association study identifies IL23R as an inflammatory bowel disease gene. *Science.* 2006;314:1461-1463.
12. Schumacher G. First attack of inflammatory bowel disease and infectious colitis. A clinical, histological and microbiological study with special reference to early diagnosis. *Scand J Gastroenterol Suppl.* 1993;198:1-24.
13. Halfvarson J, Jess T, Magnuson A, et al. Environmental factors in inflammatory bowel disease: a co-twin control study of a Swedish-Danish twin population. *Inflamm Bowel Dis.* 2006;12:925-933.
14. Loftus EV, Jr. Clinical epidemiology of inflammatory bowel disease: Incidence, prevalence, and environmental influences. *Gastroenterology.* 2004;126:1504-1517.
15. Hanauer SB. Inflammatory bowel disease: epidemiology, pathogenesis, and therapeutic opportunities. *Inflamm Bowel Dis.* 2006;12 Suppl 1:S3-9.
16. Cashman KD, Shanahan F. Is nutrition an aetiological factor for inflammatory bowel disease? *Eur J Gastroenterol Hepatol.* 2003;15:607-613.
17. Reif S, Klein I, Lubin F, Farbstein M, Hallak A, Gilat T. Pre-illness dietary factors in inflammatory bowel disease. *Gut.* 1997;40:754-760.
18. Tragnone A, Valpiani D, Miglio F, et al. Dietary habits as risk factors for inflammatory bowel disease. *Eur J Gastroenterol Hepatol.* 1995;7:47-51.
19. Dietary and other risk factors of ulcerative colitis. A case-control study in Japan. Epidemiology Group of the Research Committee of Inflammatory Bowel Disease in Japan. *J Clin Gastroenterol.* 1994;19:166-171.
20. Persson PG, Ahlbom A, Hellers G. Diet and inflammatory bowel disease: a case-control study. *Epidemiology.* 1992;3:47-52.
21. Mahmud N, Weir DG. The urban diet and Crohn's disease: is there a relationship? *Eur J Gastroenterol Hepatol.* 2001;13:93-95.
22. Amre DK, D'Souza S, Morgan K, et al. Imbalances in Dietary Consumption of Fatty Acids, Vegetables, and Fruits Are Associated With Risk for Crohn's Disease in Children. *Am J Gastroenterol.* 2007.
23. O'Sullivan M, O'Morain C. Nutrition in inflammatory bowel disease. *Best Pract Res Clin Gastroenterol.* 2006;20:561-573.
24. Glassman MS, Newman LJ, Berezin S, Gryboski JD. Cow's milk protein sensitivity during infancy in patients with inflammatory bowel disease. *Am J Gastroenterol.* 1990;85:838-840.
25. Ceyhan BB, Karakurt S, Cevik H, Sungur M. Bronchial hyperreactivity and allergic status in inflammatory bowel disease. *Respiration.* 2003;70:60-66.

26. D'Arienzo A, Manguso F, Scarpa R, et al. Ulcerative colitis, seronegative spondyloarthropathies and allergic diseases: the search for a link. *Scand J Gastroenterol.* 2002;37:1156-1163.
27. Weng X, Liu L, Barcellos LF, Allison JE, Herrinton LJ. Clustering of inflammatory bowel disease with immune mediated diseases among members of a northern california-managed care organization. *Am J Gastroenterol.* 2007;102:1429-1435.
28. D'Inca R, Annese V, di Leo V, et al. Increased intestinal permeability and NOD2 variants in familial and sporadic Crohn's disease. *Aliment Pharmacol Ther.* 2006;23:1455-1461.
29. Irvine EJ, Marshall JK. Increased intestinal permeability precedes the onset of Crohn's disease in a subject with familial risk. *Gastroenterology.* 2000;119:1740-1744.
30. Lim WC, Hanauer SB, Li YC. Mechanisms of disease: vitamin D and inflammatory bowel disease. *Nat Clin Pract Gastroenterol Hepatol.* 2005;2:308-315.
31. Froicu M, Cantorna MT. Vitamin D and the vitamin D receptor are critical for control of the innate immune response to colonic injury. *BMC Immunol.* 2007;8:5.
32. Godet PG, May GR, Sutherland LR. Meta-analysis of the role of oral contraceptive agents in inflammatory bowel disease. *Gut.* 1995;37:668-673.
33. Garcia Rodriguez LA, Gonzalez-Perez A, Johansson S, Wallander MA. Risk factors for inflammatory bowel disease in the general population. *Aliment Pharmacol Ther.* 2005;22:309-315.
34. Russell RK, Farhadi R, Wilson M, Drummond H, Satsangi J, Wilson DC. Perinatal passive smoke exposure may be more important than childhood exposure in the risk of developing childhood IBD. *Gut.* 2005;54:1500-1501; author reply 1501.
35. Mahid SS, Minor KS, Stromberg AJ, Galandiuk S. Active and passive smoking in childhood is related to the development of inflammatory bowel disease. *Inflamm Bowel Dis.* 2007;13:431-438.
36. Cosnes J. Tobacco and IBD: relevance in the understanding of disease mechanisms and clinical practice. *Best Pract Res Clin Gastroenterol.* 2004;18:481-496.
37. Sonntag B, Stolze B, Heinecke A, et al. Preterm birth but not mode of delivery is associated with an increased risk of developing inflammatory bowel disease later in life. *Inflamm Bowel Dis.* 2007.
38. Cosnes J, Seksik P, Nion-Larmurier I, Beaugerie L, Gendre JP. Prior appendectomy and the phenotype and course of Crohn's disease. *World J Gastroenterol.* 2006;12:1235-1242.
39. Reddy D, Siegel CA, Sands BE, Kane S. Possible association between isotretinoin and inflammatory bowel disease. *Am J Gastroenterol.* 2006;101:1569-1573.
40. Rolanda C, Macedo G. Isotretinoin and inflammatory bowel disease. *Am J Gastroenterol.* 2007;102:1330.
41. Mylonaki M, Langmead L, Pantes A, Johnson F, Rampton DS. Enteric infection in relapse of inflammatory bowel disease: importance of microbiological examination of stool. *Eur J Gastroenterol Hepatol.* 2004;16:775-778.
42. Rodemann JF, Dubberke ER, Reske KA, Seo da H, Stone CD. Incidence of Clostridium difficile infection in inflammatory bowel disease. *Clin Gastroenterol Hepatol.* 2007;5:339-344.
43. Issa M, Vijayapal A, Graham MB, et al. Impact of Clostridium difficile on inflammatory bowel disease. *Clin Gastroenterol Hepatol.* 2007;5:345-351.
44. Naser SA, Ghobrial G, Romero C, Valentine JF. Culture of Mycobacterium avium subspecies paratuberculosis from the blood of patients with Crohn's disease. *Lancet.* 2004;364:1039-1044.
45. Romero C, Hamdi A, Valentine JF, Naser SA. Evaluation of surgical tissue from patients with Crohn's disease for the presence of Mycobacterium avium subspecies paratuberculosis DNA by in situ hybridization and nested polymerase chain reaction. *Inflamm Bowel Dis.* 2005;11:116-125.
46. Autschbach F, Eisold S, Hinz U, et al. High prevalence of Mycobacterium avium subspecies paratuberculosis IS900 DNA in gut tissues from individuals with Crohn's disease. *Gut.* 2005;54:944-949.
47. Nakase H, Nishio A, Tamaki H, et al. Specific antibodies against recombinant protein of insertion element 900 of Mycobacterium avium subspecies paratuberculosis in Japanese patients with Crohn's disease. *Inflamm Bowel Dis.* 2006;12:62-69.
48. Polymeros D, Bogdanos DP, Day R, Arioli D, Vergani D, Forbes A. Does cross-reactivity between mycobacterium avium paratuberculosis and human intestinal antigens characterize Crohn's disease? *Gastroenterology.* 2006;131:85-96.
49. Kotlowski R, Bernstein CN, Sepehri S, Krause DO. High prevalence of Escherichia coli belonging to the B2+D phylogenetic group in inflammatory bowel disease. *Gut.* 2007;56:669-675.
50. Sasaki M, Sitaraman SV, Babbin BA, et al. Invasive Escherichia coli are a feature of Crohn's disease. *Lab Invest.* 2007.
51. Darfeuille-Michaud A, Boudeau J, Bulois P, et al. High prevalence of adherent-invasive Escherichia coli associated with ileal mucosa in Crohn's disease. *Gastroenterology.* 2004;127:412-421.
52. Martin HM, Campbell BJ, Hart CA, et al. Enhanced Escherichia coli adherence and invasion in Crohn's disease and colon cancer. *Gastroenterology.* 2004;127:80-93.
53. Heimesaat MM, Fischer A, Jahn HK, et al. Exacerbation of murine ileitis by Toll-like receptor 4 mediated sensing of lipopolysaccharide from commensal Escherichia coli. *Gut.* 2007;56:941-948.
54. Dimitroulia E, Spanakis N, Konstantinidou AE, Legakis NJ, Tsakris A. Frequent detection of cytomegalovirus in the intestine of patients with inflammatory bowel disease. *Inflamm Bowel Dis.* 2006;12:879-884.
55. Kandiel A, Lashner B. Cytomegalovirus colitis complicating inflammatory bowel disease. *Am J Gastroenterol.* 2006;101:2857-2865.
56. Saebo A, Vik E, Lange OJ, Matuszkiewicz L. Inflammatory bowel disease associated with Yersinia enterocolitica O:3 infection. *Eur J Intern Med.* 2005;16:176-182.
57. Boorom KF. Is this recently characterized gastrointestinal pathogen responsible for rising rates of inflammatory bowel disease (IBD) and IBD associated autism in Europe and the United States in the 1990s? *Med Hypotheses.* 2007;69:652-659.
58. Castiglione F, Del Vecchio Blanco G, Rispo A, et al. Orocecal transit time and bacterial overgrowth in patients with Crohn's disease. *J Clin Gastroenterol.* 2000;31:63-66.
59. Funayama Y, Sasaki I, Naito H, et al. Monitoring and antibacterial treatment for postoperative bacterial overgrowth in Crohn's disease. *Dis Colon Rectum.* 1999;42:1072-1077.
60. Castiglione F, Rispo A, Di Girolamo E, et al. Antibiotic treatment of small bowel bacterial overgrowth in patients with Crohn's disease. *Aliment Pharmacol Ther.* 2003;18:1107-1112.
61. Dassopoulos T, Frangakis C, Cruz-Correa M, et al. Antibodies to saccharomyces cerevisiae in Crohn's disease: higher titers are associated with a greater frequency of mutant NOD2/CARD15 alleles and with a higher probability of complicated disease. *Inflamm Bowel Dis.* 2007;13:143-151.

62. Konrad A, Rutten C, Flogerzi B, Styner M, Goke B, Seibold F. Immune sensitization to yeast antigens in ASCA-positive patients with Crohn's disease. *Inflamm Bowel Dis.* 2004;10:97-105.
63. Standaert-Vitse A, Jouault T, Vandewalle P, et al. Candida albicans is an immunogen for anti-Saccharomyces cerevisiae antibody markers of Crohn's disease. *Gastroenterology.* 2006;130:1764-1775.
64. Van Den Bogaerde J, Cahill J, Emmanuel AV, et al. Gut mucosal response to food antigens in Crohn's disease. *Aliment Pharmacol Ther.* 2002;16:1903-1915.
65. Jowett SL, Seal CJ, Pearce MS, et al. Influence of dietary factors on the clinical course of ulcerative colitis: a prospective cohort study. *Gut.* 2004;53:1479-1484.
66. Jones VA, Dickinson RJ, Workman E, Wilson AJ, Freeman AH, Hunter JO. Crohn's disease: maintenance of remission by diet. *Lancet.* 1985;2:177-180.
67. Jowett SL, Seal CJ, Phillips E, Gregory W, Barton JR, Welfare MR. Dietary beliefs of people with ulcerative colitis and their effect on relapse and nutrient intake. *Clin Nutr.* 2004;23:161-170.
68. Felder JB, Korelitz BI, Rajapakse R, Schwarz S, Horatagis AP, Gleim G. Effects of nonsteroidal antiinflammatory drugs on inflammatory bowel disease: a case-control study. *Am J Gastroenterol.* 2000;95:1949-1954.
69. Wilcox GM, Mattia AR. Rofecoxib and inflammatory bowel disease: clinical and pathologic observations. *J Clin Gastroenterol.* 2005;39:142-143.
70. Takeuchi K, Smale S, Premchand P, et al. Prevalence and mechanism of nonsteroidal anti-inflammatory drug-induced clinical relapse in patients with inflammatory bowel disease. *Clin Gastroenterol Hepatol.* 2006;4:196-202.
71. Evans JM, McMahon AD, Murray FE, McDevitt DG, MacDonald TM. Non-steroidal anti-inflammatory drugs are associated with emergency admission to hospital for colitis due to inflammatory bowel disease. *Gut.* 1997;40:619-622.
72. Bonner GF, Walczak M, Kitchen L, Bayona M. Tolerance of nonsteroidal antiinflammatory drugs in patients with inflammatory bowel disease. *Am J Gastroenterol.* 2000;95:1946-1948.
73. Mahadevan U, Loftus EV, Jr., Tremaine WJ, Sandborn WJ. Safety of selective cyclooxygenase-2 inhibitors in inflammatory bowel disease. *Am J Gastroenterol.* 2002;97:910-914.
74. El Miedany Y, Youssef S, Ahmed I, El Gaafary M. The gastrointestinal safety and effect on disease activity of etoricoxib, a selective cox-2 inhibitor in inflammatory bowel diseases. *Am J Gastroenterol.* 2006;101:311-317.
75. Forrest K, Symmons D, Foster P. Systematic review: is ingestion of paracetamol or non-steroidal anti-inflammatory drugs associated with exacerbations of inflammatory bowel disease? *Aliment Pharmacol Ther.* 2004;20:1035-1043.
76. Guslandi M. Exacerbation of inflammatory bowel disease by nonsteroidal anti-inflammatory drugs and cyclooxygenase-2 inhibitors: fact or fiction? *World J Gastroenterol.* 2006;12:1509-1510.
77. Bitton A, Sewitch MJ, Peppercorn MA, et al. Psychosocial determinants of relapse in ulcerative colitis: a longitudinal study. *Am J Gastroenterol.* 2003;98:2203-2208.
78. Mawdsley JE, Rampton DS. Psychological stress in IBD: new insights into pathogenic and therapeutic implications. *Gut.* 2005;54:1481-1491.
79. Hart A, Kamm MA. Review article: mechanisms of initiation and perpetuation of gut inflammation by stress. *Aliment Pharmacol Ther.* 2002;16:2017-2028.
80. Fuller-Thomson E, Sulman J. Depression and inflammatory bowel disease: findings from two nationally representative Canadian surveys. *Inflamm Bowel Dis.* 2006;12:697-707.
81. Mittermaier C, Dejaco C, Waldhoer T, et al. Impact of depressive mood on relapse in patients with inflammatory bowel disease: a prospective 18-month follow-up study. *Psychosom Med.* 2004;66:79-84.
82. Bouma G, Strober W. The immunological and genetic basis of inflammatory bowel disease. *Nat Rev Immunol.* 2003;3:521-533.
83. Imada A, Ina K, Shimada M, et al. Coordinate upregulation of interleukin-8 and growth-related gene product-alpha is present in the colonic mucosa of inflammatory bowel. *Scand J Gastroenterol.* 2001;36:854-864.
84. Jupp J, Hillier K, Elliott DH, et al. Colonic expression of leukotriene-pathway enzymes in inflammatory bowel diseases. *Inflamm Bowel Dis.* 2007;13:537-546.
85. Mudter J, Neurath MF. Il-6 signaling in inflammatory bowel disease: Pathophysiological role and clinical relevance. *Inflamm Bowel Dis.* 2007;13:1016-1023.
86. O'Connor TM, O'Connell J, O'Brien DI, Goode T, Bredin CP, Shanahan F. The role of substance P in inflammatory disease. *J Cell Physiol.* 2004;201:167-180.
87. Eivindson M, Gronbaek H, Flyvbjerg A, Frystyk J, Zimmermann-Nielsen E, Dahlerup JF. The insulin-like growth factor (IGF)-system in active ulcerative colitis and Crohn's disease: relations to disease activity and corticosteroid treatment. *Growth Horm IGF Res.* 2007;17:33-40.
88. Vagianos K, Bector S, McConnell J, Bernstein CN. Nutrition assessment of patients with inflammatory bowel disease. *JPEN J Parenter Enteral Nutr.* 2007;31:311-319.
89. Geerling BJ, Badart-Smook A, Stockbrugger RW, Brummer RJ. Comprehensive nutritional status in recently diagnosed patients with inflammatory bowel disease compared with population controls. *Eur J Clin Nutr.* 2000;54:514-521.
90. Peyrin-Biroulet L, Rodriguez-Gueant RM, Chamaillard M, et al. Vascular and cellular stress in inflammatory bowel disease: revisiting the role of homocysteine. *Am J Gastroenterol.* 2007;102:1108-1115.
91. Sturniolo GC, Fries W, Mazzon E, Di Leo V, Barollo M, D'Inca R. Effect of zinc supplementation on intestinal permeability in experimental colitis. *J Lab Clin Med.* 2002;139:311-315.
92. Sturniolo GC, Di Leo V, Ferronato A, D'Odorico A, D'Inca R. Zinc supplementation tightens "leaky gut" in Crohn's disease. *Inflamm Bowel Dis.* 2001;7:94-98.
93. Galland L. Magnesium and inflammatory bowel disease. *Magnesium.* 1988;7:78-83.
94. McConnell N, Campbell S, Gillanders I, Rolton H, Danesh B. Risk factors for developing renal stones in inflammatory bowel disease. *BJU Int.* 2002;89:835-841.
95. Giannini S, Martes C. Anemia in inflammatory bowel disease. *Minerva Gastroenterol Dietol.* 2006;52:275-291.
96. Gasche C, Lomer MC, Cavill I, Weiss G. Iron, anaemia, and inflammatory bowel diseases. *Gut.* 2004;53:1190-1197.
97. Rezaie A, Parker RD, Abdollahi M. Oxidative stress and pathogenesis of inflammatory bowel disease: an epiphenomenon or the cause? *Dig Dis Sci.* 2007;52:2015-2021.
98. Schulte CM. Review article: bone disease in inflammatory bowel disease. *Aliment Pharmacol Ther.* 2004;20 Suppl 4:43-49.
99. Bernstein CN. Inflammatory bowel diseases as secondary causes of osteoporosis. *Curr Osteoporos Rep.* 2006;4:116-123.

100. van Hogezand RA, Hamdy NA. Skeletal morbidity in inflammatory bowel disease. *Scand J Gastroenterol Suppl.* 2006:59-64.
101. Reinshagen M, Von Tirpitz C. Diagnosis and management of osteoporosis in inflammatory bowel disease. *Minerva Med.* 2004;95:481-487.
102. Droge W, Holm E. Role of cysteine and glutathione in HIV infection and other diseases associated with muscle wasting and immunological dysfunction. *Faseb J.* 1997;11:1077-1089.
103. Burnham JM, Shults J, Semeao E, et al. Body-composition alterations consistent with cachexia in children and young adults with Crohn disease. *Am J Clin Nutr.* 2005;82:413-420.
104. Moylan JS, Reid MB. Oxidative stress, chronic disease, and muscle wasting. *Muscle Nerve.* 2007;35:411-429.
105. Spate U, Schulze PC. Proinflammatory cytokines and skeletal muscle. *Curr Opin Clin Nutr Metab Care.* 2004;7:265-269.
106. Kalyani RR, Gavini S, Dobs AS. Male hypogonadism in systemic disease. *Endocrinol Metab Clin North Am.* 2007;36:333-348.
107. Anisman H, Merali Z. Cytokines, stress and depressive illness: brain-immune interactions. *Ann Med.* 2003;35:2-11.
108. Jansen G, van der Heijden J, Oerlemans R, et al. Sulfasalazine is a potent inhibitor of the reduced folate carrier: implications for combination therapies with methotrexate in rheumatoid arthritis. *Arthritis Rheum.* 2004;50:2130-2139.
109. Mason JB, Dickstein A, Jacques PF, et al. A temporal association between folic acid fortification and an increase in colorectal cancer rates may be illuminating important biological principles: a hypothesis. *Cancer Epidemiol Biomarkers Prev.* 2007;16:1325-1329.
110. Schroder O, Stein J. Low dose methotrexate in inflammatory bowel disease: current status and future directions. *Am J Gastroenterol.* 2003;98:530-537.
111. Katz JA. Treatment of inflammatory bowel disease with corticosteroids. *Gastroenterol Clin North Am.* 2004;33:171-189, vii.
112. Graff LA, Walker JR, Lix L, et al. The relationship of inflammatory bowel disease type and activity to psychological functioning and quality of life. *Clin Gastroenterol Hepatol.* 2006;4:1491-1501.
113. Persoons P, Vermeire S, Demyttenaere K, et al. The impact of major depressive disorder on the short- and long-term outcome of Crohn's disease treatment with infliximab. *Aliment Pharmacol Ther.* 2005;22:101-110.
114. Weinryb RM, Gustavsson JP, Barber JP. Personality traits predicting long-term adjustment after surgery for ulcerative colitis. *J Clin Psychol.* 2003;59:1015-1029.
115. Oliveira S, Zaltman C, Elia C, et al. Quality-of-life measurement in patients with inflammatory bowel disease receiving social support. *Inflamm Bowel Dis.* 2007;13:470-474.
116. Bernklev T, Jahnsen J, Henriksen M, et al. Relationship between sick leave, unemployment, disability, and health-related quality of life in patients with inflammatory bowel disease. *Inflamm Bowel Dis.* 2006;12:402-412.
117. Locke GR, 3rd, Zinsmeister AR, Talley NJ, Fett SL, Melton LJ, 3rd. Familial association in adults with functional gastrointestinal disorders. *Mayo Clin Proc.* 2000;75:907-912.
118. Bellentani S, Baldoni P, Petrella S, et al. A simple score for the identification of patients at high risk of organic diseases of the colon in the family doctor consulting room. The Local IBS Study Group. *Fam Pract.* 1990;7:307-312.
119. Levy RL, Whitehead WE, Von Korff MR, Feld AD. Intergenerational transmission of gastrointestinal illness behavior. *Am J Gastroenterol.* 2000;95:451-456.
120. Kalantar JS, Locke GR, 3rd, Zinsmeister AR, Beighley CM, Talley NJ. Familial aggregation of irritable bowel syndrome: a prospective study. *Gut.* 2003;52:1703-1707.
121. Levy RL, Jones KR, Whitehead WE, Feld SI, Talley NJ, Corey LA. Irritable bowel syndrome in twins: heredity and social learning both contribute to etiology. *Gastroenterology.* 2001;121:799-804.
122. Saito YA, Locke GR, 3rd, Zimmerman JM, et al. A genetic association study of 5-HTT LPR and GNbeta3 C825T polymorphisms with irritable bowel syndrome. *Neurogastroenterol Motil.* 2007;19:465-470.
123. Park JM, Choi MG, Park JA, et al. Serotonin transporter gene polymorphism and irritable bowel syndrome. *Neurogastroenterol Motil.* 2006;18:995-1000.
124. Saito YA, Petersen GM, Locke GR, 3rd, Talley NJ. The genetics of irritable bowel syndrome. *Clin Gastroenterol Hepatol.* 2005;3:1057-1065.
125. Collins SM. The relationship of enteric microbial infection and functional bowel disorders. *J Clin Gastroenterol.* 2007;41 Suppl 1:S30-32.
126. Spiller RC. Role of infection in irritable bowel syndrome. *J Gastroenterol.* 2007;42 Suppl 17:41-47.
127. Ruigomez A, Garcia Rodriguez LA, Panes J. Risk of irritable bowel syndrome after an episode of bacterial gastroenteritis in general practice: influence of comorbidities. *Clin Gastroenterol Hepatol.* 2007;5:465-469.
128. Corazziari E. Definition and epidemiology of functional gastrointestinal disorders. *Best Pract Res Clin Gastroenterol.* 2004;18:613-631.
129. Parry SD, Barton JR, Welfare MR. Factors associated with the development of post-infectious functional gastrointestinal diseases: does smoking play a role? *Eur J Gastroenterol Hepatol.* 2005;17:1071-1075.
130. Verdu EF, Bercik P, Verma-Gandhu M, et al. Specific probiotic therapy attenuates antibiotic induced visceral hypersensitivity in mice. *Gut.* 2006;55:182-190.
131. Maxwell PR, Rink E, Kumar D, Mendall MA. Antibiotics increase functional abdominal symptoms. *Am J Gastroenterol.* 2002;97:104-108.
132. Mendall MA, Kumar D. Antibiotic use, childhood affluence and irritable bowel syndrome (IBS). *Eur J Gastroenterol Hepatol.* 1998;10:59-62.
133. Gwee KA, Graham JC, McKendrick MW, et al. Psychometric scores and persistence of irritable bowel after infectious diarrhoea. *Lancet.* 1996;347:150-153.
134. Powell N, Huntley B, Beech T, Knight W, Knight H, Corrigan CJ. Increased prevalence of gastrointestinal symptoms in patients with allergic disease. *Postgrad Med J.* 2007;83:182-186.
135. Cole JA, Rothman KJ, Cabral HJ, Zhang Y, Farraye FA. Incidence of IBS in a cohort of people with asthma. *Dig Dis Sci.* 2007;52:329-335.
136. Ozol D, Uz E, Bozalan R, Turkay C, Yildirim Z. Relationship between asthma and irritable bowel syndrome: role of food allergy. *J Asthma.* 2006;43:773-775.
137. Whitehead WE, Palsson O, Jones KR. Systematic review of the comorbidity of irritable bowel syndrome with other disorders: what are the causes and implications? *Gastroenterology.* 2002;122:1140-1156.
138. Frissora CL, Koch KL. Symptom overlap and comorbidity of irritable bowel syndrome with other conditions. *Curr Gastroenterol Rep.* 2005;7:264-271.
139. Schur EA, Afari N, Furberg H, et al. Feeling bad in more ways than one: comorbidity patterns of medically unexplained and psychiatric conditions. *J Gen Intern Med.* 2007;22:818-821.
140. Cole JA, Rothman KJ, Cabral HJ, Zhang Y, Farraye FA. Migraine, fibromyalgia, and depression among people with IBS: a prevalence study. *BMC Gastroenterol.* 2006;6:26.

141. Arnold LD, Bachmann GA, Rosen R, Kelly S, Rhoads GG. Vulvodynia: Characteristics and Associations With Comorbidities and Quality of Life. *Obstet Gynecol.* 2006;107:617-624.
142. Kendall-Tackett KA. Physiological correlates of childhood abuse: chronic hyperarousal in PTSD, depression, and irritable bowel syndrome. *Child Abuse Negl.* 2000;24:799-810.
143. Katon W, Sullivan M, Walker E. Medical symptoms without identified pathology: relationship to psychiatric disorders, childhood and adult trauma, and personality traits. *Ann Intern Med.* 2001;134:917-925.
144. Walker EA, Katon WJ, Roy-Byrne PP, Jemelka RP, Russo J. Histories of sexual victimization in patients with irritable bowel syndrome or inflammatory bowel disease. *Am J Psychiatry.* 1993;150:1502-1506.
145. Evans JM, Fleming KC, Talley NJ, Schleck CD, Zinsmeister AR, Melton LJ, 3rd. Relation of colonic transit to functional bowel disease in older people: a population-based study. *J Am Geriatr Soc.* 1998;46:83-87.
146. Jarrett M, Heitkemper MM, Bond EF, Georges J. Comparison of diet composition in women with and without functional bowel disorder. *Gastroenterol Nurs.* 1994;16:253-258.
147. Malhotra S, Rana SV, Sinha SK, Khurana S. Dietary fiber assessment of patients with irritable bowel syndrome from Northern India. *Indian J Gastroenterol.* 2004;23:217-218.
148. Monsbakken KW, Vandvik PO, Farup PG. Perceived food intolerance in subjects with irritable bowel syndrome-- etiology, prevalence and consequences. *Eur J Clin Nutr.* 2006;60:667-672.
149. Lea R, Whorwell PJ. The role of food intolerance in irritable bowel syndrome. *Gastroenterol Clin North Am.* 2005;34:247-255.
150. Jun DW, Lee OY, Yoon HJ, et al. Food intolerance and skin prick test in treated and untreated irritable bowel syndrome. *World J Gastroenterol.* 2006;12:2382-2387.
151. Zar S, Mincher L, Benson MJ, Kumar D. Food-specific IgG4 antibody-guided exclusion diet improves symptoms and rectal compliance in irritable bowel syndrome. *Scand J Gastroenterol.* 2005;40:800-807.
152. Grazioli B, Matera G, Laratta C, et al. Giardia lamblia infection in patients with irritable bowel syndrome and dyspepsia: a prospective study. *World J Gastroenterol.* 2006;12:1941-1944.
153. Stark D, van Hal S, Marriott D, Ellis J, Harkness J. Irritable bowel syndrome: a review on the role of intestinal protozoa and the importance of their detection and diagnosis. *Int J Parasitol.* 2007;37:11-20.
154. Santelmann H, Howard JM. Yeast metabolic products, yeast antigens and yeasts as possible triggers for irritable bowel syndrome. *Eur J Gastroenterol Hepatol.* 2005;17:21-26.
155. Riordan SM, Kim R. Bacterial overgrowth as a cause of irritable bowel syndrome. *Curr Opin Gastroenterol.* 2006;22:669-673.
156. Pimentel M, Chow EJ, Lin HC. Normalization of lactulose breath testing correlates with symptom improvement in irritable bowel syndrome. a double-blind, randomized, placebo-controlled study. *Am J Gastroenterol.* 2003;98:412-419.
157. Parisi G, Leandro G, Bottona E, et al. Small intestinal bacterial overgrowth and irritable bowel syndrome. *Am J Gastroenterol.* 2003;98:2572; author reply 2573-2574.
158. Lupascu A, Gabrielli M, Lauritano EC, et al. Hydrogen glucose breath test to detect small intestinal bacterial overgrowth: a prevalence case-control study in irritable bowel syndrome. *Aliment Pharmacol Ther.* 2005;22:1157-1160.
159. Pimentel M, Chow EJ, Lin HC. Eradication of small intestinal bacterial overgrowth reduces symptoms of irritable bowel syndrome. *Am J Gastroenterol.* 2000;95:3503-3506.
160. Si JM, Yu YC, Fan YJ, Chen SJ. Intestinal microecology and quality of life in irritable bowel syndrome patients. *World J Gastroenterol.* 2004;10:1802-1805.
161. Malinen E, Rinttila T, Kajander K, et al. Analysis of the fecal microbiota of irritable bowel syndrome patients and healthy controls with real-time PCR. *Am J Gastroenterol.* 2005;100:373-382.
162. Madden JA, Hunter JO. A review of the role of the gut microflora in irritable bowel syndrome and the effects of probiotics. *Br J Nutr.* 2002;88 Suppl 1:S67-72.
163. Kim HJ, Vazquez Roque MI, Camilleri M, et al. A randomized controlled trial of a probiotic combination VSL# 3 and placebo in irritable bowel syndrome with bloating. *Neurogastroenterol Motil.* 2005;17:687-696.
164. Kajander K, Hatakka K, Poussa T, Farkkila M, Korpela R. A probiotic mixture alleviates symptoms in irritable bowel syndrome patients: a controlled 6-month intervention. *Aliment Pharmacol Ther.* 2005;22:387-394.
165. Nobaek S, Johansson ML, Molin G, Ahrne S, Jeppsson B. Alteration of intestinal microflora is associated with reduction in abdominal bloating and pain in patients with irritable bowel syndrome. *Am J Gastroenterol.* 2000;95:1231-1238.
166. King TS, Elia M, Hunter JO. Abnormal colonic fermentation in irritable bowel syndrome. *Lancet.* 1998;352:1187-1189.
167. Monnikes H, Tebbe JJ, Hildebrandt M, et al. Role of stress in functional gastrointestinal disorders. Evidence for stress-induced alterations in gastrointestinal motility and sensitivity. *Dig Dis.* 2001;19:201-211.
168. Bennett EJ, Tennant CC, Piesse C, Badcock CA, Kellow JE. Level of chronic life stress predicts clinical outcome in irritable bowel syndrome. *Gut.* 1998;43:256-261.
169. Hertig VL, Cain KC, Jarrett ME, Burr RL, Heitkemper MM. Daily stress and gastrointestinal symptoms in women with irritable bowel syndrome. *Nurs Res.* 2007;56:399-406.
170. Dancey CP, Taghavi M, Fox RJ. The relationship between daily stress and symptoms of irritable bowel: a time-series approach. *J Psychosom Res.* 1998;44:537-545.
171. Horwitz BJ, Fisher RS. The irritable bowel syndrome. *N Engl J Med.* 2001;344:1846 1850.
172. Mawe GM, Coates MD, Moses PL. Review article: intestinal serotonin signalling in irritable bowel syndrome. *Aliment Pharmacol Ther.* 2006;23:1067-1076.
173. Wood JD. Effects of bacteria on the enteric nervous system: implications for the irritable bowel syndrome. *J Clin Gastroenterol.* 2007;41:S7-19.
174. Guilarte M, Santos J, de Torres I, et al. Diarrhoea-predominant IBS patients show mast cell activation and hyperplasia in the jejunum. *Gut.* 2007;56:203-209.
175. Barbara G, Wang B, Stanghellini V, et al. Mast cell-dependent excitation of visceral-nociceptive sensory neurons in irritable bowel syndrome. *Gastroenterology.* 2007;132:26-37.
176. Palsson OS, Morteau O, Bozymski EM, et al. Elevated vasoactive intestinal peptide concentrations in patients with irritable bowel syndrome. *Dig Dis Sci.* 2004;49:1236-1243.

177. Akiho H, Deng Y, Blennerhassett P, Kanbayashi H, Collins SM. Mechanisms underlying the maintenance of muscle hypercontractility in a model of postinfective gut dysfunction. *Gastroenterology.* 2005;129:131-141.
178. Dinan TG, Quigley EM, Ahmed SM, et al. Hypothalamic-pituitary-gut axis dysregulation in irritable bowel syndrome: plasma cytokines as a potential biomarker? *Gastroenterology.* 2006;130:304-311.
179. Halpert A, Drossman D. Biopsychosocial issues in irritable bowel syndrome. *J Clin Gastroenterol.* 2005;39:665-669.
180. Lembo A, Ameen VZ, Drossman DA. Irritable bowel syndrome: toward an understanding of severity. *Clin Gastroenterol Hepatol.* 2005;3:717-725.
181. Schmulson MJ, Ortiz-Garrido OM, Hinojosa C, Arcila D. A single session of reassurance can acutely improve the self-perception of impairment in patients with IBS. *J Psychosom Res.* 2006;61:461-467.
182. Lackner JM, Quigley BM, Blanchard EB. Depression and abdominal pain in IBS patients: the mediating role of catastrophizing. *Psychosom Med.* 2004;66:435-441.
183. Heitkemper MM, Jarrett ME, Levy RL, et al. Self-management for women with irritable bowel syndrome. *Clin Gastroenterol Hepatol.* 2004;2:585-596.
184. Silman AJ, Pearson JE. Epidemiology and genetics of rheumatoid arthritis. *Arthritis Res.* 2002;4 Suppl 3:S265-272.
185. van der Helm-van Mil AH, Huizinga TW, de Vries RR, Toes RE. Emerging patterns of risk factor make-up enable subclassification of rheumatoid arthritis. *Arthritis Rheum.* 2007;56:1728-1735.
186. Haier J, Nasralla M, Franco AR, Nicolson GL. Detection of mycoplasmal infections in blood of patients with rheumatoid arthritis. *Rheumatology (Oxford).* 1999;38:504-509.
187. Ramirez AS, Rosas A, Hernandez-Beriain JA, et al. Relationship between rheumatoid arthritis and Mycoplasma pneumoniae: a case-control study. *Rheumatology (Oxford).* 2005;44:912-914.
188. Horowitz S, Evinson B, Borer A, Horowitz J. Mycoplasma fermentans in rheumatoid arthritis and other inflammatory arthritides. *J Rheumatol.* 2000;27:2747-2753.
189. Johnson S, Sidebottom D, Bruckner F, Collins D. Identification of Mycoplasma fermentans in synovial fluid samples from arthritis patients with inflammatory disease. *J Clin Microbiol.* 2000;38:90-93.
190. Rivera A, Yanez A, Leon-Tello G, et al. Experimental arthritis induced by a clinical Mycoplasma fermentans isolate. *BMC Musculoskelet Disord.* 2002;3:15.
191. Rashid T, Ebringer A. Rheumatoid arthritis is linked to Proteus-the evidence. *Clin Rheumatol.* 2007;26:1036-1043.
192. Rashid T, Jayakumar KS, Binder A, Ellis S, Cunningham P, Ebringer A. Rheumatoid arthritis patients have elevated antibodies to cross-reactive and non cross-reactive antigens from Proteus microbes. *Clin Exp Rheumatol.* 2007;25:259-267.
193. Oliver JE, Silman AJ. Risk factors for the development of rheumatoid arthritis. *Scand J Rheumatol.* 2006;35:169-174.
194. Jolly M, Curran JJ. Chlamydial infection preceding the development of rheumatoid arthritis: a brief report. *Clin Rheumatol.* 2004;23:453-455.
195. Singh IP, Das SK, Sharma P, Dutta GP, Agarwal SS. Antibodies to Entamoeba histolytica in patients with rheumatoid arthritis. *Trop Gastroenterol.* 1985;6:141-144.
196. Gerard HC, Wang Z, Wang GF, et al. Chromosomal DNA from a variety of bacterial species is present in synovial tissue from patients with various forms of arthritis. *Arthritis Rheum.* 2001;44:1689-1697.
197. Toivanen P. From reactive arthritis to rheumatoid arthritis. *J Autoimmun.* 2001;16:369-371.
198. Cutolo M, Sulli A, Pizzorni C, Craviotto C, Straub RH. Hypothalamic-pituitary-adrenocortical and gonadal functions in rheumatoid arthritis. *Ann N Y Acad Sci.* 2003;992:107-117.
199. Geenen R, Van Middendorp H, Bijlsma JW. The impact of stressors on health status and hypothalamic-pituitary-adrenal axis and autonomic nervous system responsiveness in rheumatoid arthritis. *Ann N Y Acad Sci.* 2006;1069:77-97.
200. Eijsbouts AM, van den Hoogen FH, Laan RF, Hermus AR, Sweep CG, van de Putte LB. Hypothalamic-pituitary-adrenal axis activity in patients with rheumatoid arthritis. *Clin Exp Rheumatol.* 2005;23:658-664.
201. Kanik KS, Wilder RL. Hormonal alterations in rheumatoid arthritis, including the effects of pregnancy. *Rheum Dis Clin North Am.* 2000;26:805-823.
202. Choi HK. Dietary risk factors for rheumatic diseases. *Curr Opin Rheumatol.* 2005;17:141-146.
203. Benito-Garcia E, Feskanich D, Hu FB, Mandl LA, Karlson EW. Protein, iron, and meat consumption and risk for rheumatoid arthritis: a prospective cohort study. *Arthritis Res Ther.* 2007;9:R16.
204. Merlino LA, Curtis J, Mikuls TR, Cerhan JR, Criswell LA, Saag KG. Vitamin D intake is inversely associated with rheumatoid arthritis: results from the Iowa Women's Health Study. *Arthritis Rheum.* 2004;50:72-77.
205. Grant WB. Epidemiology of disease risks in relation to vitamin D insufficiency. *Prog Biophys Mol Biol.* 2006;92:65-79.
206. Ponsonby AL, Lucas RM, van der Mei IA. UVR, vitamin D and three autoimmune diseases--multiple sclerosis, type 1 diabetes, rheumatoid arthritis. *Photochem Photobiol.* 2005;81:1267-1275.
207. Pedersen LM, Permin H. Rheumatic disease, heavy-metal pigments, and the Great Masters. *Lancet.* 1988;1:1267-1269.
208. Klareskog L, Padyukov L, Alfredsson L. Smoking as a trigger for inflammatory rheumatic diseases. *Curr Opin Rheumatol.* 2007;19:49-54.
209. Severijnen AJ, Kool J, Swaak AJ, Hazenberg MP. Intestinal flora of patients with rheumatoid arthritis: induction of chronic arthritis in rats by cell wall fragments from isolated Eubacterium aerofaciens strains. Br J Rheumatol. 1990;29:433-439.
210. Haugen MA, Kjeldsen-Kragh J, Skakkebaek N, et al. The influence of fast and vegetarian diet on parameters of nutritional status in patients with rheumatoid arthritis. Clin Rheumatol. 1993;12:62-69; Kjeldsen-Kragh J, Haugen M, Borchgrevink CF, et al. Controlled trial of fasting and one-year vegetarian diet in rheumatoid arthritis. Lancet. 1991;338:899-902.
211. Kjeldsen-Kragh J, Mellbye OJ, Haugen M, et al. Changes in laboratory variables in rheumatoid arthritis patients during a trial of fasting and one-year vegetarian diet. Scand J Rheumatol. 1995;24:85-93.
212. Kjeldsen-Kragh J. Rheumatoid arthritis treated with vegetarian diets. Am J Clin Nutr. 1999;70:594S-600S.
213. Kjeldsen-Kragh J, Hvatum M, Haugen M, Forre O, Scott H. Antibodies against dietary antigens in rheumatoid arthritis patients treated with fasting and a one-year vegetarian diet. Clin Exp Rheumatol. 1995;13:167-172.
214. Rashid T, Darlington G, Kjeldsen-Kragh J, Forre O, Collado A, Ebringer A. Proteus IgG antibodies and C-reactive protein in English, Norwegian and Spanish patients with rheumatoid arthritis. Clin Rheumatol. 1999;18:190-195.
215. Finckh A, Iversen M, Liang MH. The exercise prescription in rheumatoid arthritis: primum non nocere. *Arthritis Rheum.* 2003;48:2393-2395.

216. Pool AJ, Whipp BJ, Skasick AJ, Alavi A, Bland JM, Axford JS. Serum cortisol reduction and abnormal prolactin and CD4+/CD8+ T-cell response as a result of controlled exercise in patients with rheumatoid arthritis and systemic lupus erythematosus despite unaltered muscle energetics. *Rheumatology (Oxford).* 2004;43:43-48.
217. Case JP. Old and new drugs used in rheumatoid arthritis: a historical perspective. Part 1: the older drugs. *Am J Ther.* 2001;8:123-143.
218. Toh ML, Miossec P. The role of T cells in rheumatoid arthritis: new subsets and new targets. *Curr Opin Rheumatol.* 2007;19:284-288.
219. Szekanecz Z, Koch AE. Macrophages and their products in rheumatoid arthritis. *Curr Opin Rheumatol.* 2007;19:289-295.
220. Brennan F, Beech J. Update on cytokines in rheumatoid arthritis. *Curr Opin Rheumatol.* 2007;19:296-301.
221. Eklund KK. Mast cells in the pathogenesis of rheumatic diseases and as potential targets for anti-rheumatic therapy. *Immunol Rev.* 2007;217:38-52.
222. Rosenstein ED, Caldwell JR. Trace elements in the treatment of rheumatic conditions. *Rheum Dis Clin North Am.* 1999;25:929-935, viii.
223. Tuncer S, Kamanli A, Akcil E, Kavas GO, Seckin B, Atay MB. Trace element and magnesium levels and superoxide dismutase activity in rheumatoid arthritis. *Biol Trace Elem Res.* 1999;68:137-142.
224. Kremer JM, Bigaouette J. Nutrient intake of patients with rheumatoid arthritis is deficient in pyridoxine, zinc, copper, and magnesium. *J Rheumatol.* 1996;23:990-994.
225. Agrawal S, Misra R, Aggarwal A. Anemia in rheumatoid arthritis: high prevalence of iron-deficiency anemia in Indian patients. *Rheumatol Int.* 2006;26:1091-1095.
226. Wilson A, Yu HT, Goodnough LT, Nissenson AR. Prevalence and outcomes of anemia in rheumatoid arthritis: a systematic review of the literature. *Am J Med.* 2004;116 Suppl 7A:50S-57S.
227. Hitchon CA, El-Gabalawy HS. Oxidation in rheumatoid arthritis. *Arthritis Res Ther.* 2004;6:265-278.
228. Sinigaglia L, Varenna M, Girasole G, Bianchi G. Epidemiology of osteoporosis in rheumatic diseases. *Rheum Dis Clin North Am.* 2006;32:631-658.
229. Walsmith J, Roubenoff R. Cachexia in rheumatoid arthritis. *Int J Cardiol.* 2002;85:89-99.
230. Isik A, Koca SS, Ozturk A, Mermi O. Anxiety and depression in patients with rheumatoid arthritis. *Clin Rheumatol.* 2007;26:872-878.
231. Schiepers OJ, Wichers MC, Maes M. Cytokines and major depression. *Prog Neuropsychopharmacol Biol Psychiatry.* 2005;29:201-217.
232. Whittle SL, Hughes RA. Folate supplementation and methotrexate treatment in rheumatoid arthritis: a review. *Rheumatology (Oxford).* 2004;43:267-271.
233. Conn DL, Lim SS. New role for an old friend: prednisone is a disease-modifying agent in early rheumatoid arthritis. *Curr Opin Rheumatol.* 2003;15:193-196.
234. Groarke A, Curtis R, Coughlan R, Gsel A. The role of perceived and actual disease status in adjustment to rheumatoid arthritis. *Rheumatology (Oxford).* 2004;43:1142-1149.
235. Edwards RR, Bingham CO, 3rd, Bathon J, Haythornthwaite JA. Catastrophizing and pain in arthritis, fibromyalgia, and other rheumatic diseases. *Arthritis Rheum.* 2006;55:325-332.
236. Treharne GJ, Lyons AC, Booth DA, Kitas GD. Psychological well-being across 1 year with rheumatoid arthritis: coping resources as buffers of perceived stress. *Br J Health Psychol.* 2007;12:323-345.
237. Zautra AJ, Parrish BP, Van Puymbroeck CM, et al. Depression history, stress, and pain in rheumatoid arthritis patients. *J Behav Med.* 2007;30:187-197.
238. Holtzman S, Delongis A. One day at a time: The impact of daily satisfaction with spouse responses on pain, negative affect and catastrophizing among individuals with rheumatoid arthritis. *Pain.* 2007;131:202-213.
239. Buskila D, Neumann L. Fibromyalgia syndrome (FM) and nonarticular tenderness in relatives of patients with FM. *J Rheumatol.* 1997;24:941-944.
240. Arnold LM, Hudson JI, Hess EV, et al. Family study of fibromyalgia. *Arthritis Rheum.* 2004;50:944-952.
241. Buskila D. Genetics of chronic pain states. *Best Pract Res Clin Rheumatol.* 2007;21:535-547.
242. Ablin JN, Cohen H, Buskila D. Mechanisms of Disease: genetics of fibromyalgia. *Nat Clin Pract Rheumatol.* 2006;2:671-678.
243. Tishler M, Smorodin T, Vazina-Amit M, Ramot Y, Koffler M, Fishel B. Fibromyalgia in diabetes mellitus. *Rheumatol Int.* 2003;23:171-173.
244. Cleveland CH, Jr., Fisher RH, Brestel EP, Esinhart JD, Metzger WJ. Chronic rhinitis: an underrecognized association with fibromyalgia. *Allergy Proc.* 1992;13:263-267.
245. Tuncer T, Butun B, Arman M, Akyokus A, Doseyen A. Primary fibromyalgia and allergy. *Clin Rheumatol.* 1997;16:9-12.
246. Sinaii N, Cleary SD, Ballweg ML, Nieman LK, Stratton P. High rates of autoimmune and endocrine disorders, fibromyalgia, chronic fatigue syndrome and atopic diseases among women with endometriosis: a survey analysis. *Hum Reprod.* 2002;17:2715-2724.
247. Ablin JN, Shoenfeld Y, Buskila D. Fibromyalgia, infection and vaccination: Two more parts in the etiological puzzle. *J Autoimmun.* 2006;27:145-152.
248. Cairns V, Godwin J. Post-Lyme borreliosis syndrome: a meta-analysis of reported symptoms. *Int J Epidemiol.* 2005;34:1340-1345.
249. Nasralla M, Haier J, Nicolson GL. Multiple mycoplasmal infections detected in blood of patients with chronic fatigue syndrome and/or fibromyalgia syndrome. *Eur J Clin Microbiol Infect Dis.* 1999;18:859-865.
250. Endresen GK. Mycoplasma blood infection in chronic fatigue and fibromyalgia syndromes. *Rheumatol Int.* 2003;23:211-215.
251. Adak B, Tekeoglu I, Ediz L, et al. Fibromyalgia frequency in hepatitis B carriers. *J Clin Rheumatol.* 2005;11:157-159.
252. Douche-Aourik F, Berlier W, Feasson L, et al. Detection of enterovirus in human skeletal muscle from patients with chronic inflammatory muscle disease or fibromyalgia and healthy subjects. *J Med Virol.* 2003;71:540-547.
253. L. Galland ML, H. Bueno, C Heirnowitz. Giardia lamblia infection as a cause of chronic fatigue. *Journal of Nutritional Medicine.* 1990;2:27-32.
254. Galland L. Patient-centered diagnosis and treatment for chronic fatigue syndrome. *American Academy of Environmental Medicine Annual Scientific Session.* Virginia Beach, VA; 1994.
255. Levine PH, Jacobson S, Pocinki AG, et al. Clinical, epidemiologic, and virologic studies in four clusters of the chronic fatigue syndrome. *Arch Intern Med.* 1992;152:1611-1616.
256. Tanriverdi F, Karaca Z, Unluhizarci K, Kelestimur F. The hypothalamo-pituitary-adrenal axis in chronic fatigue syndrome and fibromyalgia syndrome. *Stress.* 2007;10:13-25.
257. Huisman AM, White KP, Algra A, et al. Vitamin D levels in women with systemic lupus erythematosus and fibromyalgia. *J Rheumatol.* 2001;28:2535-2539.
258. Armstrong DJ, Meenagh GK, Bickle I, Lee AS, Curran ES, Finch MB. Vitamin D deficiency is associated with anxiety and depression in fibromyalgia. *Clin Rheumatol.* 2007;26:551-554.
259. McLean SA, Williams DA, Clauw DJ. Fibromyalgia after motor vehicle collision: evidence and implications. *Traffic Inj Prev.* 2005;6:97-104.

260. Hughes L. Physical and psychological variables that influence pain in patients with fibromyalgia. *Orthop Nurs.* 2006;25:112-119; quiz 120-111.
261. Seng JS, Graham-Bermann SA, Clark MK, McCarthy AM, Ronis DL. Posttraumatic stress disorder and physical comorbidity among female children and adolescents: results from service-use data. *Pediatrics.* 2005;116:e767-776.
262. Van Houdenhove B, Neerinckx E, Onghena P, Lysens R, Vertommen H. Premorbid "overactive" lifestyle in chronic fatigue syndrome and fibromyalgia. An etiological factor or proof of good citizenship? *J Psychosom Res.* 2001;51:571-576.
263. Aaron LA, Buchwald D. Chronic diffuse musculoskeletal pain, fibromyalgia and co-morbid unexplained clinical conditions. *Best Pract Res Clin Rheumatol.* 2003;17:563-574.
264. Ifergane G, Buskila D, Simiseshvely N, Zeev K, Cohen H. Prevalence of fibromyalgia syndrome in migraine patients. *Cephalalgia.* 2006;26:451-456.
265. Tietjen GE, Bushnell CD, Herial NA, Utley C, White L, Hafeez F. Endometriosis is associated with prevalence of comorbid conditions in migraine. *Headache.* 2007;47:1069-1078.
266. Carta MG, Cardia C, Mannu F, et al. The high frequency of manic symptoms in fibromyalgia does influence the choice of treatment? *Clin Pract Epidemol Ment Health.* 2006;2:36.
267. Kato K, Sullivan PF, Evengard B, Pedersen NL. Chronic widespread pain and its comorbidities: a population-based study. *Arch Intern Med.* 2006;166:1649-1654.
268. Staud R. Are patients with systemic lupus erythematosus at increased risk for fibromyalgia? *Curr Rheumatol Rep.* 2006;8:430-435.
269. Bazzichi L, Rossi A, Giuliano T, et al. Association between thyroid autoimmunity and fibromyalgic disease severity. *Clin Rheumatol.* 2007.
270. Garrison RL, Breeding PC. A metabolic basis for fibromyalgia and its related disorders: the possible role of resistance to thyroid hormone. *Med Hypotheses.* 2003;61:182-189.
271. Haugen M, Kjeldsen-Kragh J, Nordvag BY, Forre O. Diet and disease symptoms in rheumatic diseases--results of a questionnaire based survey. *Clin Rheumatol.* 1991;10:401-407.
272. Smith JD, Terpening CM, Schmidt SO, Gums JG. Relief of fibromyalgia symptoms following discontinuation of dietary excitotoxins. *Ann Pharmacother.* 2001;35:702-706.
273. Miller CS. The compelling anomaly of chemical intolerance. *Ann N Y Acad Sci.* 2001;933:1-23.
274. Pimentel M, Wallace D, Hallegua D, et al. A link between irritable bowel syndrome and fibromyalgia may be related to findings on lactulose breath testing. *Ann Rheum Dis.* 2004;63:450-452.
275. Cater RE, 2nd. Chronic intestinal candidiasis as a possible etiological factor in the chronic fatigue syndrome. *Med Hypotheses.* 1995;44:507-515.
276. Hickie I, Davenport T, Wakefield D, et al. Post-infective and chronic fatigue syndromes precipitated by viral and non-viral pathogens: prospective cohort study. *Bmj.* 2006;333:575.
277. Seet RC, Quek AM, Lim EC. Post-infectious fatigue syndrome in dengue infection. *J Clin Virol.* 2007;38:1-6.
278. Ledina D, Bradaric N, Milas I, Ivic I, Brncic N, Kuzmicic N. Chronic fatigue syndrome after Q fever. *Med Sci Monit.* 2007;13:CS88-92.
279. Machtey I. Chlamydia pneumoniae antibodies in myalgia of unknown cause (including fibromyalgia). *Br J Rheumatol.* 1997;36:1134.
280. Vierck CJ, Jr., Staud R, Price DD, Cannon RL, Mauderli AP, Martin AD. The effect of maximal exercise on temporal summation of second pain (windup) in patients with fibromyalgia syndrome. *J Pain.* 2001;2:334-344.
281. Kosek E, Ekholm J, Hansson P. Modulation of pressure pain thresholds during and following isometric contraction in patients with fibromyalgia and in healthy controls. *Pain.* 1996;64:415-423.
282. Staud R, Robinson ME, Price DD. Isometric exercise has opposite effects on central pain mechanisms in fibromyalgia patients compared to normal controls. *Pain.* 2005;118:176-184.
283. Jones KD, Clark SR. Individualizing the exercise prescription for persons with fibromyalgia. *Rheum Dis Clin North Am.* 2002;28:419-436, x-xi.
284. Okifuji A, Turk DC. Stress and psychophysiological dysregulation in patients with fibromyalgia syndrome. *Appl Psychophysiol Biofeedback.* 2002;27:129-141.
285. Martinez-Lavin M. Biology and therapy of fibromyalgia. Stress, the stress response system, and fibromyalgia. *Arthritis Res Ther.* 2007;9:216.
286. Abeles AM, Pillinger MH, Solitar BM, Abeles M. Narrative review: the pathophysiology of fibromyalgia. *Ann Intern Med.* 2007;146:726-734.
287. Ozgocmen S, Ozyurt H, Sogut S, Akyol O. Current concepts in the pathophysiology of fibromyalgia: the potential role of oxidative stress and nitric oxide. *Rheumatol Int.* 2006;26:585-597.
288. Wood PB, Schweinhardt P, Jaeger E, et al. Fibromyalgia patients show an abnormal dopamine response to pain. *Eur J Neurosci.* 2007;25:3576-3582.
289. Russell IJ, Orr MD, Littman B, et al. Elevated cerebrospinal fluid levels of substance P in patients with the fibromyalgia syndrome. *Arthritis Rheum.* 1994;37:1593-1601.
290. Bazzichi L, Rossi A, Massimetti G, et al. Cytokine patterns in fibromyalgia and their correlation with clinical manifestations. *Clin Exp Rheumatol.* 2007;25:225-230.
291. Salemi S, Rethage J, Wollina U, et al. Detection of interleukin 1beta (IL-1beta), IL-6, and tumor necrosis factor-alpha in skin of patients with fibromyalgia. *J Rheumatol.* 2003;30:146-150.
292. Regland B, Andersson M, Abrahamsson L, Bagby J, Dyrehag LE, Gottfries CG. Increased concentrations of homocysteine in the cerebrospinal fluid in patients with fibromyalgia and chronic fatigue syndrome. *Scand J Rheumatol.* 1997;26:301-307.
293. Moorkens G, Manuel y Keenoy B, Vertommen J, Meludu S, Noe M, De Leeuw I. Magnesium deficit in a sample of the Belgian population presenting with chronic fatigue. *Magnes Res.* 1997;10:329-337.
294. Galland L. Magnesium and immune function: an overview. *Magnesium.* 1988;7:290-299.
295. Turk DC, Robinson JP, Burwinkle T. Prevalence of fear of pain and activity in patients with fibromyalgia syndrome. *J Pain.* 2004;5:483-490.
296. Garcia-Campayo J, Pascual A, Alda M, Gonzalez Ramirez MT. Coping with fibromialgia: Usefulness of the Chronic Pain Coping Inventory-42. *Pain.* 2007.
297. Schleicher H, Alonso C, Shirtcliff EA, Muller D, Loevinger BL, Coe CL. In the face of pain: the relationship between psychological well-being and disability in women with fibromyalgia. *Psychother Psychosom.* 2005;74:231-239.
298. Crooks VA. Exploring the altered daily geographies and lifeworlds of women living with fibromyalgia syndrome: a mixed-method approach. *Soc Sci Med.* 2007;64:577-588.

Chapter 5

Clinical Applications: Applying Functional Medicine to Gut Dysregulation

The conventional, disease-centered approach described in Chapter 3 views each ailment as a discrete entity classified according to an ICD code. Functional medicine, in contrast, views health and illness as a continuum along which all components of the human biological system interact dynamically with the environment to produce patterns that change over time in the individual. The functional medicine approach moves from the 20th century focus on *organ system medicine* to a 21st century methodology for clinical application of the evolving concepts of *systems biology medicine*. Gut dysfunction can be assessed and managed extremely well with this emerging model.

To manage the complexity inherent in this approach, functional medicine has adopted 2 practical models that lead to individualized, patient-centered therapies. Chapter 4 introduced and illustrated the essential concepts of antecedent conditions, triggering events, and mediators of dysfunctional processes underlying classical diagnoses of disease. In this chapter, we will introduce the *Functional Medicine Matrix Model* (see Figure 5.2), a tool for collecting, sorting, and prioritizing a vast amount of clinical information in a rigorous, disciplined process. Clinical case studies of fibromyalgia, rheumatoid arthritis, irritable bowel syndrome, and inflammatory bowel disease will be presented to demonstrate this method of integrating the *antecedents-triggers-mediators* model within the clinical algorithms of functional medicine and the matrix.

Core Clinical Imbalances and the Functional Medicine Matrix Model

The practice of functional medicine is characterized by an examination of the *core clinical imbalances* that underlie the expression of disease. Those imbalances arise as a result of insufficiencies or excesses in diet, individual nutrients, exercise, exposure to various toxic influences, or physical and emotional trauma. These exposures and "inputs" are then processed through a unique set of genetic and metabolic predispositions, attitudes, and beliefs. The core clinical imbalances that can arise involve:

- Immune surveillance
- Inflammatory process
- Oxidative-reductive homeodynamics
- Digestion, absorption, and barrier integrity (these gastrointestinal factors can also include microbiological imbalances)
- Detoxification and biotransformation
- Structural integrity (from cellular membrane function to the musculoskeletal system)
- Hormonal and neurotransmitter regulation
- Psychological and spiritual equilibrium

When imbalances in these areas develop, we see them as precursors to the signs and symptoms from which conventionally trained practitioners detect and label (diagnose) organ system disease. These imbalances arise from dysfunctions or defects within the fundamental physiological and psychological processes that cut across all organ systems; they alert the functional medicine practitioner to pay attention to the full expression of dysfunction and disease. Each of these imbalances is explored in considerable detail in the *Textbook of Functional Medicine,*[1] where the underlying evidence supporting this approach to patient care is thoroughly discussed. In *Section VII: Putting It All Together* of the textbook, there are extensive chapters reviewing, through step-by-step illustrations, the methodologies and heuristics of functional medicine. The most important precept to remember about functional medicine is that restoring balance—in the patient's environmental inputs and in the body's fundamental physiological processes—is the preeminent activity in both evaluating and treating chronic illness and in improving health. Restoring balance involves much more than treating symptoms. Functional medicine requires a disciplined, critical mind that asks the basic clinical questions, what were the *antecedent conditions* that engendered a susceptibility to *triggering events*, and what are the *mediators* and *processes of mediation* of the ongoing dis-eased condition(s)?

Figure 5.1 illustrates the integration of the antecedents-triggers-mediators model and the Functional Medicine Matrix Model. The matrix provides a comprehensive methodology for rigorously pursuing relevant patient information required for comprehensive assessment and therapeutic plan development. A basic principle of functional medicine is biochemical individuality and environmental uniqueness; practitioners must evaluate each patient's unique set of antecedents, triggers, mediators, and signs and symptoms in order to create an individualized treatment plan. Because a human being is an interconnected web and not just a potpourri of discrete organ systems, all the input should be examined for patterns, interconnections, and points of leverage. That is what the matrix helps us do, in a shorthand way.

Arrow #1: Patient Signs and Symptoms: The Therapeutic Encounter and the Narrative

The first step in the patient encounter requires diligent history taking and assessments. Patient information gathering includes both the subjective experiences of the patient (symptoms) and objective observations of the patient, through lab or imaging assessments and through observations by the clinician. The domain of relevant information is much larger in the context of functional medicine because the sorting system (antecedents-triggers-mediators model and Functional Medicine Matrix Model) allows for the patient's total experience to be relevant to the therapeutic encounter.

Rapport is the core element that enables a practitioner to glean the necessary information from patients. In order to listen to and understand the patient's story, help people make beneficial changes, and create a healing context, it is important to be able to develop a rapid and powerful rapport with patients so that they feel comfortable telling their stories and revealing intimate information and significant events. Collecting all the pieces of the patient's history to effectively guide assessment and treatment requires skills, training, practice, and good tools.

Healthcare practitioners—whether modern or ancient, from Western or Eastern disciplines, physician or shaman—have always needed a system for constructing an explanatory story of the patient's illness. These systems can vary from a few questions and much observation (an approach characteristic of the Yupik shaman), or prolonged palpation of the pulse while listening to the breathing pattern (a Tibetan healer), to patient questionnaires accompanied by physical exam and laboratory data (the Western medical model). Whatever the tradition or training, the healer/healthcare practitioner and patient together construct a story. The most comprehensive methods integrate experiences, perceptions, observations, and objective information into a coherent, culturally sensitive narrative. Two important outcomes are generated from a comprehensive patient story: (1) the patient is understood within a context that is often considerably broader than the standard biomedical portrait, and (2) hope is established in the minds of both patient and practitioner that steps can be taken to change the trajectory of the present illness back

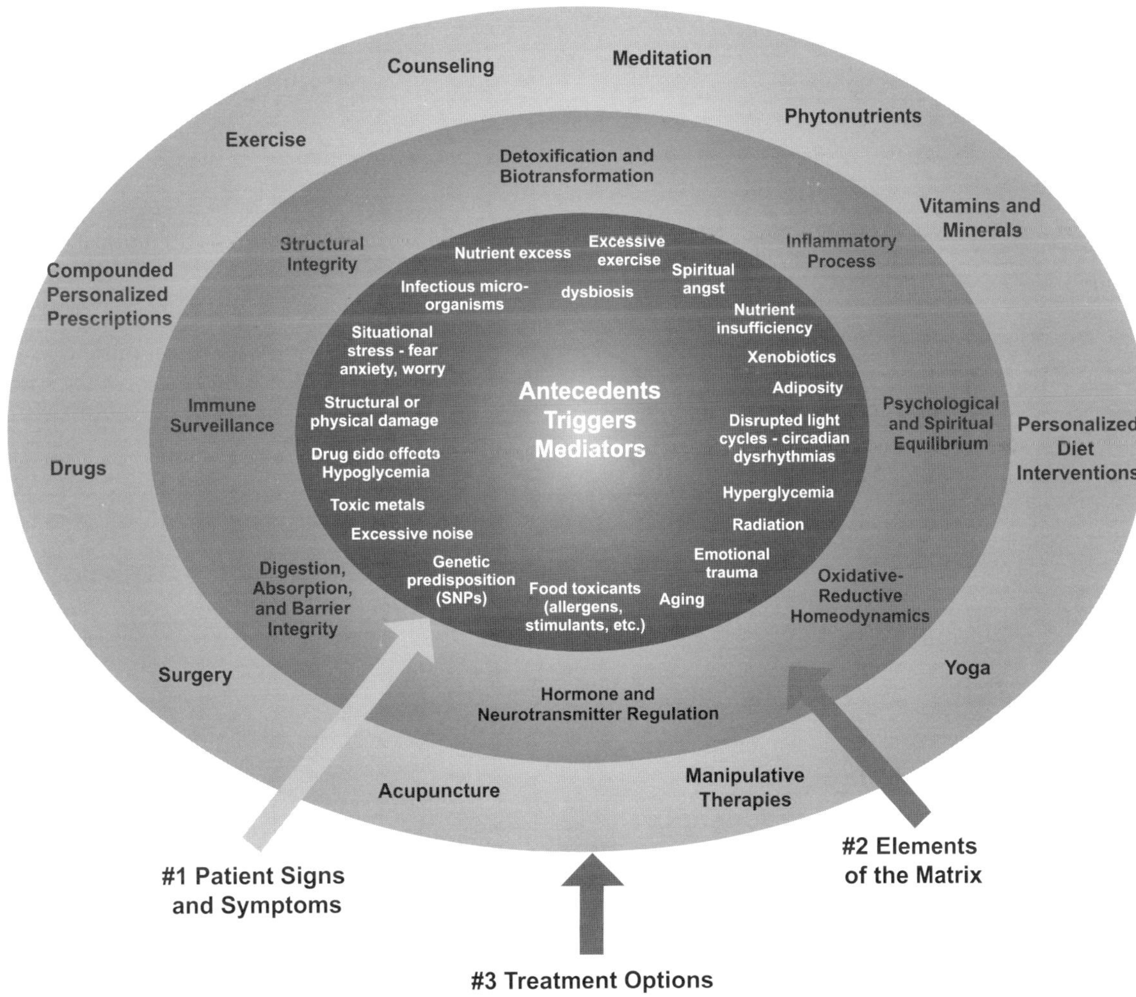

Figure 5.1—The Functional Medicine Methodology

toward health. Clinical medicine really begins with the patient's story, so it is worth our time to be sure we construct that story in a way that is appropriate to the patient, to his or her complaint(s), and to the therapeutics that can be most helpful.

Most healthcare systems have a heuristic approach to this challenge—a shorthand way of directing attention that does not require continuous application of the entire detailed decision model at every step of the process. Collecting, sorting, and focusing relevant data toward the development of a coherent story and well-founded therapeutic plan can, indeed, be cumbersome and time-consuming in the absence of an efficient model. In standard medical care, efficiency is gained by generating and sorting information through a well-established and very useful model (see Table 5.1). This standard medical heuristic is organized to distill the patient's story into a "short list" of potential diagnoses. The process of selecting among those potential diagnoses (working through the differential diagnosis) is usually facilitated by collecting further data (physical examination, laboratory measures) related to the most likely choices.

Table 5.1—Standard History and Physical

- Chief Complaint
- History of Present Illness
- Past Medical History
- Review of Organ Systems
- Family History
- Dietary History
- Medication and Supplement History
- Social, Lifestyle, and Exercise History
- Physical Exam Findings
- Laboratory and Imaging Evaluations
- Assessment and Diagnosis

The inherent goal in this conventional model is to narrow the inquiry down as quickly as possible to a specific diagnosis[2] with the expectation that such a process leads fairly directly to a therapeutic plan of (usually) pharmaceutical and/or surgical intervention(s).[3] Implicit in such a model is a belief that enough of the patient's full story can be captured by a diagnosis that an appropriate and effective treatment plan can be based upon it. The organization of information into only those categories that help the clinician formulate the diagnosis and the treatment plan simplifies the process of "doctoring" and lends coherence and reproducibility to the standard medical approach.

The cost, however, of the speed and efficiency of this conventional model is that the narrow focus precludes a comprehensive response to some of today's most common and costly conditions: chronic, complex illnesses.[4] Speed and efficiency are highly desirable in the acute care setting; however, the steady and disturbing rise in the incidence and prevalence of serious chronic diseases and the failures of the conventional model to adequately enfold the unique mixture of comorbidities into a robust portrait of the patient's medical needs beg for a more comprehensive architecture in the non-acute circumstances of chronic illnesses.

Functional medicine stands on the very substantial shoulders of the standard medical paradigm, expanding it with an emphasis on principles, mechanisms, and influences of illness that weld together meaning and mechanistic explanations to the diagnosis. The functional medicine architecture deepens the clinician's understanding of the often overlapping ways human functioning goes wrong and what to do about it. At the heart of this heuristic is the antecedents-triggers-mediators model presented previously (see Chapter 4). We now move to the next step in the heuristic of functional medicine: the Functional Medicine Matrix Model.

Arrow #2: Elements of the Matrix

Any methodology for constructing a coherent story and an effective therapeutic plan in the context of complex, chronic illness must be flexible and adaptive. Like an accordion file that can compress and expand on demand, the amount and kind of data needed will necessarily change in accordance with the patient's situation and the clinician's time and ability to piece together the underlying threads of dysfunction. In the acute setting, the clinical information requirements contract to a very slim, survival-driven set of points that provide guidance and milestones with as little extraneous information as possible in order to achieve rapid diagnosis and intervention. Relevant examples of the clinical conditions responsive to this model abound: cardiac arrest, gram-negative shock, pneumonia, herpetic corneal infection, spinal cord compression.

However, in the clinical approach to chronic illness, with multiple comorbidities, the accordion file must expand to incorporate a much larger database of relevant information. For example, the compilation of the "present illness" section of the history and physical must expand to include a thorough investigation of antecedents, triggers, and mediators if the completed story is to develop and sustain a robust partnership between the patient and the health-care provider (see Table 5.2). Personalized medical care without this essential investigation will fall short. There are many pathways that can lead to chronic, diagnosable disease; the story elements must broaden sufficiently to comprehensively assess these.[4] Diagnosis is only one step in the functional medicine process; it is not, as it often is in the standard paradigm, the final step before intervention.

Table 5.2—Functional Medicine Approach to History and Physical

- Chief Complaint
- History of Present Illness
  - ANTECEDENTS, TRIGGERS, AND MEDIATORS
- Past Medical History
- Review of Organ Systems
- Family History
- Dietary History
- Medication and Supplement History
- Social, Lifestyle, and Exercise History
- Physical Exam Findings
- Laboratory and Imaging Evaluations
- Diagnosis
  - FUNDAMENTAL CLINICAL IMBALANCES UNDERLYING THE DIAGNOSES

Functional medicine offers an approach to the comprehensive *review of essential elements and mechanisms of disease* that incorporates the rich science on the biochemistry and physiology of the human system. Also taken into account is the emerging understanding of the interaction of outside influences with internal human physiology, including the evolving body of science embedded in mind/body research. Explicit in the principles of functional medicine is the concept that each patient comprises his or her own "universe" with a unique set of interconnections, potentials, diversities, and reserve capacities.[5] Also recognized is that "the body can only be understood as a whole."[6] The functional medicine principles (see Section II of the *Textbook of Functional Medicine*[1]) add a significant level of complexity to the clinical thinking process, requiring not only more data collection but also a conscious synthesizing process: Who is this patient, both in detail and in whole?

IFM has developed specific tools to facilitate the sorting process as well as analysis/synthesis. The central organizing tool is the Functional Medicine Matrix Model. Figure 5.1 and Figure 5.2 present the same concept in 2 different formats. Figure 5.1 is a graphic that illustrates the concepts of how information flows from the initial gathering, through the processes of information sorting, to the final selection of therapies. Figure 5.2 is the clinical tool that has been developed by The Institute for Functional Medicine (IFM) for the sorting process. The information that has been gathered is distributed into the areas under each of the 8 elements of the matrix. During the process of sorting, key pieces of information will also be seen as essential to understanding the antecedent conditions that predisposed to the illnesses, and other information will emerge in the winnowing process as key to understanding how the disorder under investigation was triggered.

Distilling the data from the history, physical exam, and laboratory into a narrative story line that includes antecedents, triggers, and mediators can be daunting. As discussed above, the key to developing a thorough narrative is viewing the story through the lens of the matrix, which facilitates organizing the story according to a set of 8 common underlying influences on health. Let's investigate these 8 influences further.

1. **Immune Surveillance:** Immune imbalances have an obvious role in gastrointestinal inflammation, as well as autoimmune diseases such as rheumatoid arthritis, ankylosing spondylitis, and systemic lupus erythematosus. While the standard medical approach to this pathophysiology has focused almost exclusively on the pharmacological

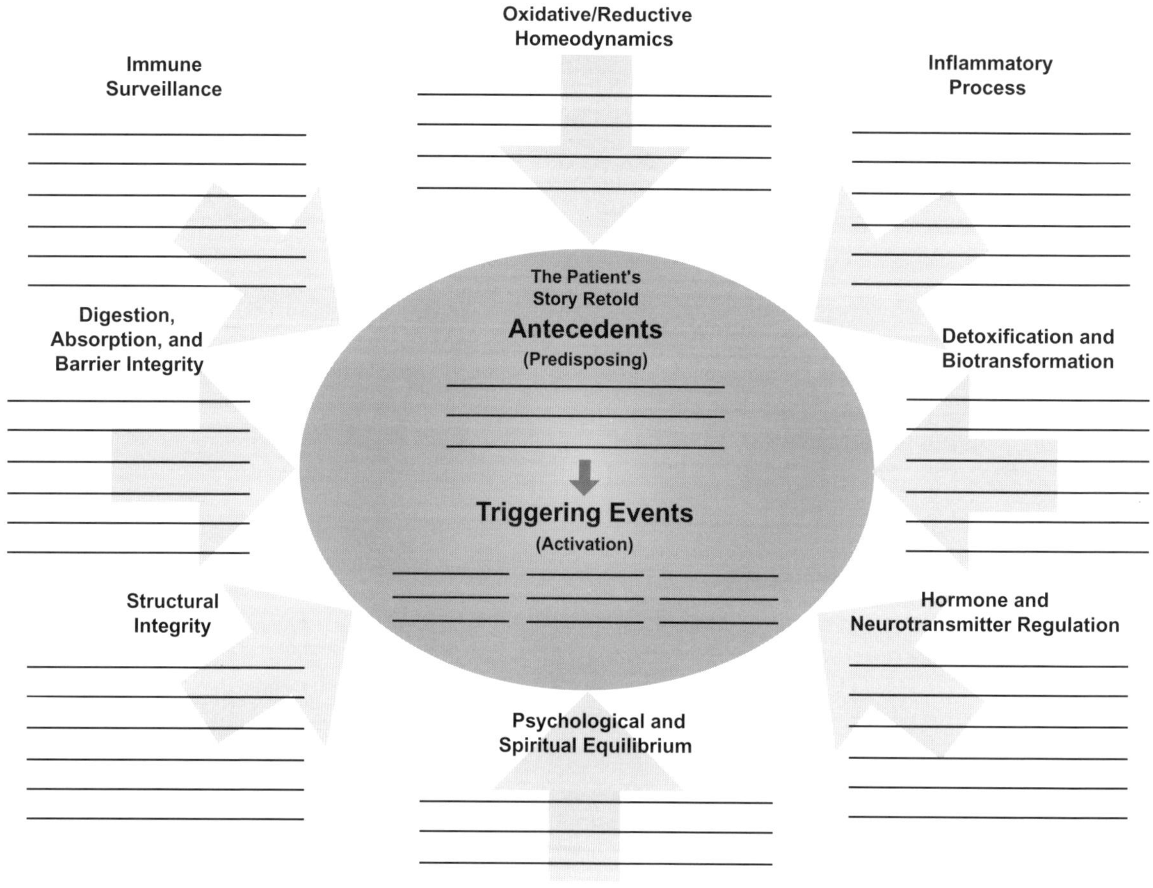

Figure 5.2—The Functional Medicine Matrix Model

suppression of resultant inflammation and tissue destruction, functional medicine has emphasized the importance of determining and addressing the underlying causes of the inherent immune imbalance. Clinicians of all disciplines must appreciate the role of pharmacological immunosuppression in the treatment of acute, inflammatory exacerbations. However, they should also appreciate that the sole reliance on immunosuppression for long-term management of immunologically mediated disorders can result in therapeutic failure insofar as it does not correct the underlying cause of the disease and creates dependency upon perpetual immunosuppression, with its attendant costs and potential for adverse effects, including infection and increased risk for cancer.

Rather than presuming that immune dysfunction and the resultant inflammation and autoimmunity are results of spontaneous generation, functional medicine clinicians seek to identify and correct the causes of these immune imbalances (when possible). In this way, clinicians can lessen or obviate the need for chronic, polypharmaceutical treatment with anti-inflammatory and immunosuppressive agents. The scientific basis of functional medicine suggests that secondary immune imbalances (distinguished from primary genetic disorders) generally arise from 1 or more of 5 main problems: (1) habitual consumption of a proinflammatory diet, (2) food allergies and intolerances, (3) microbial dysbiosis, including multifocal poly-dysbiosis, (4) hormonal imbalances, and (5) xenobiotic exposure and accumulation resulting in immunotoxicity via bystander activation and enhanced processing of autoantigens, as well as haptenization and neoantigen formation.[7] These influences may act singularly or, when combined, may be additive and synergistic. Many of these antecedents to the triggering of immune dysregulation have been discussed in this monograph.

2. Inflammatory Process: Inflammatory imbalances may be distinguished from immune imbalances insofar as inflammatory imbalances connote disorders of inflammatory mediator production in the absence of the immunodysfunction typical of allergy, autoimmunity, or immunosuppression. Here again, long-term consumption of a proinflammatory diet[8] is considered a primary trigger because the standard American diet typically oversupplies inflammatory precursors such as arachidonate and undersupplies anti-inflammatory phytonutrients such as vitamin D, zinc, selenium, and the numerous phytochemicals that reduce activation of inflammatory pathways.[9-12]

Three of the best examples of correctable inflammatory imbalances are those due to vitamin D deficiency, fatty acid imbalances, and overconsumption of simple sugars and saturated fats.

- Vitamin D deficiency is a serious health problem that spans nearly all geographic regions and socioeconomic strata. Adverse effects include systemic inflammation[13] and chronic musculoskeletal pain,[14] which both resolve quickly upon correction of the nutritional deficiency.
- Overconsumption of arachidonic acid along with underconsumption of alpha-linolenic acid (ALA), gamma-linolenic acid (GLA), eicosapentaenoic acid (EPA), docosahexaenoic acid (DHA), and oleic acid subtly yet powerfully shift nutrigenomic tendency and precursor availability in favor of enhanced systemic inflammation. Correction of this imbalance has consistently proven to be of significant clinical value in the management of chronic inflammatory disorders.[15, 16]
- Measurable increases in systemic inflammation and oxidative stress follow glucose challenge,[17] consumption of saturated fatty acids as found in cream,[18] and consumption of fast food breakfasts, which trigger the prototypic inflammatory activator nuclear factor-kappa B (NF-κB) for enhanced production of inflammatory mediators.[19]

This triad (vitamin D deficiency, fatty acid imbalance, and overconsumption of sugars and saturated fats) is typical of the Western/American pattern of dietary intake, and the molecular means and clinical consequences of such dietary choices are quite clear, evidenced by burgeoning epidemics of metabolic and inflammatory diseases.

3. Oxidative-Reductive Homeodynamics: Oxidative stress results from chronic, systemic inflammation as seen in painful disorders such as inflammatory bowel disease and rheumatoid arthritis, as well as most neurodegenerative disorders. This imbalance contributes to the perpetuation and exacerbation of inflammatory diseases via expedited tissue destruction, alterations in gene transcription, and resultant enhanced inflammatory mediator production.[20] Immune activation increases production of reactive oxygen species (free radicals). Oxidative stress increases activation of proinflammatory transcription factors and increases spontaneous oxidative modification of anatomic tissue (e.g., tissue damage and changes seen in ulcerative colitis). Thus, a vicious cycle of oxidation and inflammation exacerbates and perpetuates various inflammation-associated diseases, resulting in therapeutic recalcitrance and autonomous disease progression.[21, 22]

A rational clinical approach to breaking this vicious, pathogenic cycle can include simultaneous antioxidation and immunomodulation, the former with diet optimization and nutritional supplementation and the latter with allergen avoidance, hormonal correction, xenobiotic detoxification, balancing of gastrointestinal dysbiosis with the appropriate *4R interventions* (see Appendix), and specific *phytonutritional* modulation of proinflammatory pathways. Severe and acute inflammation can and often should be suppressed pharmacologically, but sole reliance on pharmacological immunosuppression leaves the patient vulnerable to iatrogenic immunosuppression and the well-known increased risk for cardiovascular disease, infection, and clinical malignancy; in addition, this reliance fails to address the biochemical and immunologic imbalances that underlie all chronic inflammatory and autoimmune diseases.

The contribution of mitochondrial dysfunction and increased oxidative stress is seen in a diverse group of diseases, including many with attendant recurrent or persistent pain such as migraine and fibromyalgia. In fibromyalgia, as discussed in Chapter 3, numerous abnormalities in cellular bioenergetics are noted, which correlate clinically with the lowered lactate threshold, persistent muscle pain, reduced functional capacity, and subjective fatigue that characterize the disorder.[23] Nutritional preservation and enhancement of mitochondrial function generally include, in addition to diet and lifestyle modification, supplementation with coenzyme Q10, niacin, riboflavin, thiamin, lipoic acid, magnesium, and other nutrients and botanical medicines that enhance production of adenosine triphosphate (ATP).[24]

4. Digestion, Absorption, and Barrier Integrity: The alimentary tract, its accessory organs of the liver, gallbladder, and pancreas, and the gut-associated lymphoid tissue (GALT) are often the sites of key clinical imbalances. As we have seen in this monograph, microbiological imbalances (gastrointestinal dysbiosis) are also an important and frequent clinical consideration. Impaired digestion begins neither in the stomach nor in the mouth, but it starts rather in any socioeconomic milieu that deprives people of the means to prepare wholesome, health-promoting meals and the time to consume those meals in a relaxed, parasympathetic-dominant mode. Poor dentition, xerostomia, hypochlorhydria, cholestasis or cholecystectomy, pancreatic insufficiency, mucosal atrophy, altered gut motility, and bacterial overgrowth of the small bowel are important and common contributors to impaired digestion and absorption; clinicians should consider these frequently and implement treatment with a low threshold for intervention.

Consumption of foods to which the individual is sensitized (food allergies) can trigger migraine and other chronic headaches,[25, 26] as well as generalized musculoskeletal pain and arthritis.[27-29] Avoidance of the offending foods results in amelioration or complete remission of the painful syndrome at low cost and high efficacy without reliance on expensive or potentially harmful or addictive pain-relieving drugs. As we have seen, gluten enteropathy (celiac disease) can present with arthritic pain and chronic synovitis; the pain and inflammation remit on a gluten-free diet.[30]

Alterations in intestinal microbial balance or an individual's unique response to endogenous bacteria (i.e., dysbiosis) can lead to systemic inflammation. Clinicians should appreciate that dysbiosis can occur at sites other than the gastrointestinal tract, most importantly the nasopharynx and genitourinary tracts. Eradication of the occult infection or mucosal colonization often results in marked reductions in systemic inflammation and its clinical complications.

5. Detoxification and Biotransformation: As our environment becomes increasingly polluted and as researchers and clinicians mature and expand their appreciation and knowledge of the adverse effects of xenobiotics (toxic metals and chemicals), healthcare providers will need to attend to their patients' detoxification capacity and xenobiotic load as a component of the prevention and treatment of disease. Functional medicine clinicians are aware of the association with xenobiotics in prototypic diseases such as Parkinson's disease,[31, 32] adult-onset diabetes mellitus,[33-36] and attention-deficit hyperactivity disorder.[37-39] The role of xenobiotic exposure and impaired detoxification in inflammatory disorders is more subtle and is generally mediated through the resultant immunotoxicity that manifests as autoimmunity. The numerous roles of xenobiotic exposure in the genesis and perpetuation of chronic health problems and the role of clinical detoxification in the treatment of such problems have been detailed elsewhere by Crinnion,[40-44] Rea,[45] Bland,[46, 47] Vasquez,[7, 48] and others.[49, 50]

6. Structural Integrity: Molecular structural imbalances lie at the heart of the concept of *biochemical individuality*, originated by Roger J. Williams[51] in 1956 and soon thereafter expanded into the theory and practice of *orthomolecular medicine* pioneered by Linus Pauling and colleagues.[52, 53] Pauling is considered by many authorities to be the original source of the concept of molecular medicine because he coined the phrase *molecular disease* after his team's discovery in 1949 that sickle cell anemia resulted from a single amino acid substitution that caused physical deformation of the hemoglobin molecule in hypoxic conditions.[54]

The scientific rationale for nutritional therapy is derived in part from the recognition that altered enzymatic function due to altered enzyme structure can often be corrected by administration of supra-dietary doses of nutrients. Relatedly, the structure and function of cell membranes are determined by their composition, which is influenced by dietary intake of fatty acids and which influences production of prostaglandins and leukotrienes. This is an important aspect of the scientific rationale for the use of specific fatty acid supplements in the prevention and treatment of inflammatory disease. Cell membrane structure and function can also be altered by systemic oxidative stress; the concomitant alterations in intracellular ions (e.g., calcium) and receptor function, along with activation of transcription factors such as NF-κB, contribute to widespread physiological impairment, which creates a vicious cycle of inflammation, metabolic disturbance, and additional free radical generation.[55, 56]

Somatic dysfunction, musculoskeletal disorders, and inefficient biomechanics contribute to clinically relevant disorders, as well. Physicians trained in clinical biomechanics and physical medicine appreciate the subtle nuances of musculoskeletal structure-function relationships and address these problems directly with physical and manual means rather than ignoring the physical problem and treating only its biochemical sequelae with pharmaceutical interventions.

7. Hormonal and Neurotransmitter Regulation: Hormonal imbalances are particularly relevant to the discussion of chronic inflammatory gastrointestinal disorders, characteristic of a broad group of autoimmune diseases such as inflammatory bowel disease and the arthritides. Often clinically subtle but nonetheless of extreme importance, these hormonal influences on painful inflammation are worthy of their own detailed investigation. Generally speaking and with a few noted exceptions (such as Sjögren's syndrome), the research literature points to a specific pattern of hormonal imbalances among patients with autoimmunity, and this pattern is consistent with the proinflammatory and immunodysregulatory effects of estrogens and prolactin and the anti-inflammatory and immunomodulatory effects of cortisol, dehydroepiandrosterone (DHEA), and testosterone. Appropriate therapeutic correction of these imbalances can safely result in disease amelioration.[7]

8. Psychological and Spiritual Equilibrium: The connections between inflammatory disorders, including those of gastrointestinal function, and psycho-emotional status and events are worthy of thorough investigation. A survey of the literature makes clear the interconnected nature of inflammation, psycho-emotional stress, depression, social isolation, and nutritional status. Stressful and depressive life events promote the development, persistence, and exacerbation of disorders of pain and inflammation through nutritional, hormonal, immunologic, oxidative, and microbiological mechanisms. Stated most simply, the perception of stressful events and the resultant neurohormonal cascade result in expedited metabolic utilization and increased urinary excretion of nutrients (e.g., tryptophan and zinc, magnesium, and retinol, respectively), which sum to affect nutritional imbalances and depletion, particularly when the stress response is acute or prolonged.[57-59] Stress increases secretion of prolactin, a hormone that plays an important pathogenic role in chronic inflammation and autoimmunity.[60, 61]

An abundance of experimental and clinical research supports the model that chronic psycho-emotional stress reduces mucosal immunity, increases gastrointestinal permeability, and allows for increased intestinal colonization by microbes. These microbes then stimulate immune responses that cross-react with musculoskeletal tissues and result in the clinical manifestation of autoimmunity and painful rheumatic syndromes, which appear clinically as variants of acute and chronic reactive arthritis (formerly Reiter' syndrome[62]) in susceptible patients.[7, 63-69] Intestinal bacteria have been shown to become more virulent when their host is stressed, whereas previously these same bacteria may have been incapable of causing disease.[70, 71] Psycho-emotional stress also reduces mucosal immunity and increases colonization in locations other than the gastrointestinal tract.

Arrow #3: *Treatment Options*

In Figure 5.1, the third arrow points to therapies, which should be chosen for their potential impact on the most central imbalances of the particular patient. Evaluating interventions that are available at each of the 8 elements of the Functional Medicine Matrix Model can help to identify a reasonably comprehensive set of options from which to choose.

The initial functional medicine therapeutic approach involves foundational recommendations that produce a positive impact on multiple systems. We must answer the questions of how and where to begin (prioritization) with a particular patient. Looking for the simplest interventions that will achieve maximum impact is a reasonable starting point. Although these initial interventions may sound very basic, patients are typically quite pleased to find that implementation can produce a dramatic enhancement of well-being.

It is clear that daily behaviors, including diet and physical activity, have a large impact on health. For example, lifestyle changes have been shown to meaningfully outperform metformin in generating a higher rate of diabetes prevention.[72, 73] Secondary prevention of myocardial infarction has also been demonstrated dramatically by dietary interventions involving omega-3 fatty acids in the GISSI Trial,[74] the DART Study,[75] and the Lyon Study.[76] The functional medicine style of practice teaches patients that their daily choices have a powerful effect on their health. Therefore, in-office patient education (a very important, albeit basic, intervention) is a critical factor in achieving success with lifestyle changes. The functional medicine model requires active patient participation and may be challenging for those expecting passive delivery of health care through a prescription or surgical procedure.[77]

Numerous lifestyle modifications of benefit to the patient are likely to be identified early in a functional medicine workup. Many such changes are already familiar to most patients as recommended healthy practices, but they have not been adopted for a variety of possible reasons: unpreparedness for change, belief that low-tech interventions are unlikely to have a measurable effect, insufficient understanding of how lifestyle habits affect health, and home or work situations with little support for changing behaviors. When a practitioner or patient educator thoroughly and nonjudgmentally explains the basis for lifestyle recommendations relative to the individual's specific situation, a door opens for patients to meaningfully reevaluate their daily actions.

Patients need information, instruction, and ongoing support as they integrate untried practices and abandon comfortable habits that have long undermined their health. An integral element of the art of practicing functional medicine is the ability to encourage patients without overwhelming them. An overzealous functional medicine practitioner or educator may impair the therapeutic relationship by mandating too many changes simultaneously, when a given patient may already be struggling to put new principles into operation.

As functional medicine practitioners, we know that poor diet, toxic overload, and overstimulation of inflammatory mediators impair proper function. Consistent application of healthier lifestyle habits optimizes broad areas of function by minimizing metabolic demand. When we restore nutrient adequacy, reduce toxic burden, and diminish excessive activation of the hypothalamic-pituitary-adrenal (HPA) axis, metabolic efficiency is more likely to normalize. Patients who have been effectively instructed on these concepts often establish early improvement of symptoms before more specific and advanced interventions are suggested.

With this short overview of the integration of the antecedents-triggers-mediators model and the Functional Medicine Matrix Model, let's now move to case studies about patients with conventional diagnoses whose health was improved by this functional medicine methodology. It is not possible to describe in detail the critical thinking pathways involved in the transitions from (1) information gathering to (2) sorting of the clinical information into the relevant 8 elements of the matrix, and (3) establishing the important antecedent conditions and triggering events. A shorthand technique will be used throughout the case studies presented below. The elements of the matrix will appear in parentheses with the abbreviation *EM* for elements of the matrix (e.g., EM: GI, Inflammation); antecedents, triggers, and mediators also will appear in parentheses (e.g., ATM: dysbiosis). This shortcut will be less disruptive to the flow of the clinical narrative.

Case Reports

Fibromyalgia

SW is a 52-year-old schoolteacher with a 4-year history of diffuse muscle aching, fatigue, and non-restful sleep with gradual onset. Review of systems indicated intermittent diarrhea and abdominal pain (EM: GI) and a gradual

40-pound weight gain over the past decade (EM: Inflammation). Family history was positive for depression, migraine headaches, and mitral valve prolapse. Initial laboratory testing revealed mildly elevated erythrocyte sedimentation rate (ESR), 32 mm/h, and C-reactive protein (CRP), 4.8 mg/L (EM: Inflammation), as well as negative Lyme ELISA, rheumatoid factor, and antinuclear antibodies. Physical examination revealed numerous tender points, consistent with the American College of Rheumatology criteria for fibromyalgia. Her primary physician referred her to a rheumatologist who rendered a diagnosis of fibromyalgia and prescribed amitriptyline. The medication decreased diarrhea but increased fatigue and had no effect on pain.

For 2 years, she treated her symptoms with ibuprofen as needed. After 2 years of illness, she developed a low-grade fever and consulted an infectious disease specialist, who made a diagnosis of Lyme and bartonellosis diseases spread by the *Ixodes scapularis* tick (ATM: Infectious Agent), based upon a positive Western blot for *Borrelia* antibodies and the presence of antibodies to *Bartonella henselae* (EM: Inflammation, Immune). She was treated with various oral and intravenous antibiotics over the next 18 months. While on antibiotics, she experienced an increase in energy and decrease in pain and diarrhea, but she would relapse within 60 days of their discontinuation (ATM: Dysbiosis). Her relapses were so discouraging that she stopped working.

She consulted another infectious disease specialist, who tested her stool, which was positive for *Giardia lamblia* antigen (ATM: Infectious Agent). A 7-day course of metronidazole relieved all her symptoms for about 60 days, as had most other antibiotics. Colonoscopy performed after discontinuation of metronidazole was normal, except for the presence of diverticulosis in the descending and sigmoid colon. Following colonoscopy, she had return of all symptoms, including abdominal pain and low-grade fever (ATM: Dysbiosis).

At this point, she sought a functional medicine consultation. On physical examination, she was obese, had numerous muscular tender points, diffuse nodularity of her breasts, and generalized abdominal tenderness with voluntary guarding and rebound tenderness referred to the left lower quadrant. On laboratory testing, her ESR was 54 mm/h and her CRP was 8.7 mg/L. Total white blood cell count was 8500. The clinical diagnosis of diverticulitis was confirmed with an abdominal CT scan (EM: GI, inflammation).

Placing her acute illness in the context of her chronic ailment, I suspected that fibromyalgia may actually have been a systemic response to chronic or recurrent diverticulitis, which would explain her response to antibiotics but lack of cure (EM: GI, Immune).

I elected to treat her with rifaximin, a nonabsorbed antibiotic effective for the treatment of diverticulitis. If her response to rifaximin was inferior to her response to systemically active medication, my theory would be disproven. Rifaximin was no less effective at relieving fibromyalgia symptoms than the best of the medications prescribed for the Lyme/*Bartonella* infection. She was therefore started on a maintenance program for control of chronic diverticulitis. The goal was to control large bowel inflammation with diet and dietary supplements. The program consisted of an anti-inflammatory diet, high in fiber, phytonutrients, and omega-3 fats and designed to promote hormonal balance,[78] supplemented with (1) 20 g/d of pure vegetable cellulose, (2) *Boswellia serrata* extract, 450 mg three times a day, shown to be as effective as mesalamine in ulcerative colitis, (3) a probiotic supplying 100 trillion colony-forming units twice a day, and (4) concentrated aloe vera mucopolysaccharides, 10 g/d. Following this regimen she lost 30 pounds over the next 6 months and maintained the remission initiated by rifaximin until the time of this writing (2 years). She has returned to work full time.

This patient is presented as an example of chronic intestinal inflammation (EM: GI, Inflammation) due to colonic diverticulitis producing a systemic illness characterized by fibromyalgia and fatigue. The patient's prior response to multiple antibiotics indicated the likely presence of microbial triggers as the main factors provoking systemic inflammation (symptoms at a distance from the primary site of insult). Although refractory Lyme disease was possible, the documented episode of diverticulitis and response to a nonabsorbed antibiotic laid the basis for a successful treatment regimen for fibromyalgia based solely upon control of colonic diverticular inflammation.

Rheumatoid Arthritis

AL, a 38-year-old female real estate agent, had experienced symmetrical pain and swelling of the joints of her knees and of the metacarpophalangeal and proximal interphalangeal joints of her hands and diffuse pain and swelling of her feet for 2 years (EM: Inflammation). The symptoms had appeared over a 3-month period following marital separation (ATM: Separation). Review of systems was significant for perennial allergic rhinitis, intermittent asthma since childhood (EM: Inflammation, Immune), chronic constipation (EM: GI), and difficulty losing the weight she had gained with her first pregnancy. She was taking levothyroxine for hypothyroidism associated with Hashimoto's thyroiditis (EM: Hormonal, Immune). Prior testing had revealed allergies to dust and molds (EM: Immune). Her maternal aunt suffered from rheumatoid arthritis and her mother and sister from thyroid disease. Family history was also positive for coronary artery disease in both parents. She consulted a rheumatologist, who made a diagnosis of rheumatoid arthritis, which was confirmed by cyclic citrullinated peptide-IgG antibodies and a high titer for rheumatoid factor. Her ESR was 68 mm/h (EM: Inflammation). Nonsteroidal anti-inflammatory drugs (NSAIDs) gave her moderate relief of symptoms but caused epigastric pain and worsened constipation. She refused methotrexate because of fear of side effects. Hydroxychloroquine taken over a 3-month period produced no improvement. Her physical therapist referred her for a functional medicine consultation.

On physical examination, she had soft tissue swelling and tenderness of all metacarpophalangeal and proximal interphalangeal joints of hands and feet with decreased grip strength. There was synovial thickening and decreased range of motion of both wrists. Her knees were enlarged, warm, and fluctuant, with tenderness on palpation of the femoral-tibial joints bilaterally. Her nasal mucosa was cyanotic and edematous, consistent with allergic rhinitis. On laboratory testing, her ESR was 72 mm/h and CRP was 21.6 mg/L. She had elevated IgG and IgA antibodies to gliadin with a negative antibody response to tissue transglutaminase. Gastrointestinal permeability based on lactulose and mannitol excretion after a challenge was elevated, with a lactulose-mannitol ratio of 0.13 (EM: GI). Stool culture grew *Proteus mirabilis* in high yield with an absence of *Lactobacillus* species (ATM: Dysbiosis).

I viewed the diagnosis of rheumatoid arthritis to be accurate but incomplete. This patient had allergies, including a possible sensitivity to gluten (EM: Immune), inflammation of the small intestine, probably due to her use of NSAIDs (EM: GI; ATM: NSAIDs), and colonic dysbiosis reflected in the absence of *Lactobacillus* and heavy growth of *Proteus* in stool. *Proteus* species contain antigens that cross-react with HLA-DR4, an autoantigen associated with rheumatoid arthritis. She had become ill following a major life stress (EM: Psycho-Spiritual, Hormonal). Patients with rheumatoid arthritis and several other autoimmune diseases have been shown to have suboptimal regulation of the HPA axis with impaired cortisol secretion in response to stress, a characteristic that has been linked to subsequent development of chronic inflammation (EM: Hormonal, Inflammation). This understanding led to a multi-pronged therapeutic approach.

Discontinuation of enteropathic NSAIDs and replacement with an anti-inflammatory diet and supplements were the first steps in therapy. The patient was instructed in a diet designed to promote hormonal balance,[78] achieving a reduction in saturated fat to less than 10% of calories and a dietary omega-3-to-omega-6 ratio of 1:4, which is 3 to 5 times higher than the usual North American diet. She was advised to avoid glutinous grains (wheat, rye, barley) and mold-containing foods (primarily cheeses and fermented foods). In addition:

- The diet was supplemented with fish oil supplying 4000 mg/d of omega-3 fatty acids and borage oil supplying 1500 mg/d of GLA, each of which has been shown to have NSAID-sparing effects in patients with rheumatoid arthritis.
- For healing her small intestine, she was prescribed two powders, one containing glutamine, which has been shown to prevent NSAID enteropathy,[79] and one containing vitamins, minerals, amino acids, bioflavonoids, and the phytonutrients rutin, curcuminoids, and quercetin to nutritionally support healthy essential fatty acid metabolism.
- For reversal of dysbiosis, she was given a probiotic containing 3 species of *Lactobacillus*, at a dose of 60 billion colony-forming units a day, and the antimicrobial herb *Coptis chinensis*, which contains the alkaloid berberine, at a dose of 400 mg of berberine twice a day; berberine is effective against a range of intestinal pathogens.

The patient felt that she had adapted well to her divorce over the 3 years since separating from her husband, and she was not interested in psychotherapy or stress management. Assessment of adrenal function was deferred until her response to the nutritional regimen could be ascertained.

The diet change produced a decline in pain and swelling of all joints within 7 days. Over the next 6 months, she lost 24 pounds, returning to her pre-pregnancy weight, and experienced further reduction in signs and symptoms of arthritis, so that her only symptom was mild morning stiffness of her hands and feet. Her ESR declined to 24 mm/h and her CRP to 1.9 mg/L. Once her gastrointestinal permeability had become normal, the glutamine supplement was discontinued. When repeat stool testing showed no growth of *Proteus* species, *Coptis chinensis* was discontinued.

The principles of treatment for this patient are quite similar to the principles of treatment in the first case study, even though one patient has classic rheumatoid arthritis and the other fibromyalgia. The main difference is that the patient with rheumatoid arthritis needed a more restricted diet and a more stringent anti-inflammatory program because of the severity of inflammation and the presence of allergy.

Irritable Bowel Syndrome

JK, a 34-year-old male construction worker, sought a functional medicine approach to treatment of gastrointestinal complaints of 5 years' duration. His initial symptom had been severe epigastric pain, traced to the presence of *Helicobacter pylori* gastritis (ATM: Infectious Agent). Triple therapy with bismuth, amoxicillin, and clarithromycin eliminated this symptom but left him with heartburn and belching. Upper gastrointestinal endoscopy revealed cure of *H. pylori* with the development of a new problem—gastroesophageal reflux. He was given a series of proton pump inhibitors (PPIs), which relieved the heartburn but led to the onset of new symptoms, including cramping lower abdominal pain, distension, flatulence, and frequent loose bowel movements (EM: GI). He observed that fasting reduced symptoms, and eating almost any meal increased them; in addition, antibiotics taken for sinus infections aggravated the symptoms (ATM: Dysbiosis).

His gastroenterologist made a clinical diagnosis of small bowel bacterial overgrowth and administered rifaximin, which made his symptoms worse. The specialist changed his diagnosis to irritable bowel syndrome and recommended vagolytics (which aggravated heartburn) and psyllium, which increased distension and flatulence. The patient tried various probiotic preparations. Some produced mild symptom relief, but those containing lactose produced symptom exacerbation (ATM: Lactose Intolerance). A hydrogen breath test following lactose challenge was definitive for lactase deficiency, and he was started on a lactose-free diet, which at best produced a 20% improvement in symptoms.

His history, more than any laboratory test, suggested the real dynamics of his illness. Neither lactose intolerance nor an intestinal motility disorder were at the root of his problems. He had become ill while suppressing gastric acid (ATM: Hypochlorhydria) with PPIs and experienced aggravation of symptoms with antibacterial therapy (EM: GI, Inflammation). Upper gastrointestinal microbial overgrowth is a documented side effect of gastric acid suppression, and the adverse response to antibiotics suggested that yeasts were the principle organisms involved in the likely dysbiosis. Stool examination supported the hypothesis. Microscopic examination revealed numerous budding yeasts that failed to grow on culture. This phenomenon, described as the presence of dead fecal yeast, has been associated with antibiotic-induced, antifungal-responsive diarrhea. It has the following explanation: stool culture has a much greater sensitivity than microscopic examination for *Candida* and related yeasts. When yeasts are seen but fail to grow on culture, they are likely to be damaged by a host defense factor, as yet unidentified; its presence indicates that in this particular patient *Candida* is not acting as a mere commensal in the gut. In a controlled but unpublished study conducted in the 1980s, I determined that patients with dead fecal yeast secreted a factor in rectal mucus that actively inhibited the growth of *Candida* on culture. This factor was confined to patients with dead yeast. A candidate for the factor is *Candida*-specific secretory IgA, which has been negatively associated with the growth of fecal yeasts.

Proof of this theory would require empirical therapy for intestinal yeast overgrowth and restoration of normal gastric acidity. For yeast control, the following steps were taken: (1) restriction of dietary sugars that are a substrate for yeast growth, (2) antifungal medication, in this case nystatin, and (3) probiotics. For restoration of normal gastric acidity, calcium citrate powder after each meal was substituted for PPIs, which are a highly unphysiological treatment for gastroesophageal reflux. They do not actually prevent reflux; they convert acid reflux to non-acid reflux. Calcium on the other hand enhances esophageal acid clearance and increases tone of the lower esophageal sphincter; calcium also has the added advantage of slowing colonic motility. Although mistakenly used as antacids, calcium salts have no measurable effect on esophageal pH. This therapeutic strategy (the integrated form of this therapeutic formalism is called the *4R program*—see appendix) resulted in marked reduction in all symptoms over a period of 3 weeks, which has been sustained for 18 months as of this writing. Nystatin was discontinued after 3 months, and the dietary restriction on monosaccharides was lessened shortly thereafter.

Inflammatory Bowel Disease

HB, a 27-year-old male policeman, had been given a diagnosis of Crohn's disease at the age of 22. His initial symptom had been perianal pain, traced to the presence of a rectal fissure. He soon developed diarrhea and right lower quadrant abdominal pain. He had a family history of Crohn's disease and psoriasis (EM: GI, Immune, Inflammation). Laboratory testing had shown an ESR that ranged from 36 to 75 mm/h and a chronic low-grade anemia. Review of systems indicated fluctuating fatigue, fever, and joint pains, symptoms that varied with the reactivity of his gastrointestinal symptoms (EM: GI). At colonoscopy, he was found to have ileitis and patchy colitis with a colorectal fistula. Several medications were administered in succession. Metronidazole improved his rectal fissure but caused a neuropathy and was discontinued. Mesalamine worsened diarrhea and caused hair loss. Remicade closed his anal fissure but did not affect his other symptoms. Numerous probiotics increased his symptoms. The most effective medication was prednisone, which decreased fever, pain, and diarrhea, but he was unable to reduce the dose below 15 mg (EM: GI, Immune). Azathioprine was started and discontinued because of pancreatitis.

When he came for a functional medicine consultation, his symptoms were continuous right lower quadrant pain, frequent loose bowel movements containing blood and mucus, and moderate fatigue. On physical examination, he was pale and underweight with right lower quadrant abdominal tenderness, guarding, and fullness. Laboratory studies showed a white blood cell count of 11,500, hemoglobin of 10.9 g/dL, ESR of 96 mm/h, CRP of 13.7 mg/L, and reduction in serum albumen (3.2 g/L), plasma zinc (497 mg/L), 25-hydroxy vitamin D3 (12 mcg/L) (ATM, Nutritional Insufficiency/Deficiency), and DHEA-S (37 mg/L) (ATM: Hormonal Suppression). All these deficits are the result of chronic inflammation, but some may contribute to complications of inflammatory bowel disease. Low zinc may impair growth and tissue repair; low DHEA-S and 25-hydroxy vitamin D3 are associated with bone loss. His levels of 1,25-dihydroxy vitamin D were elevated at 124 pg/L, consistent with the effect of Th1 activation on vitamin D metabolism. This patient had progressive active Crohn's disease with few conventional therapeutic options remaining.

Diet can be an effective therapy for Crohn's disease, and studies with enteral feedings have indicated that deep fistulating disease and ileitis respond best (EM: GI, Immune). Controlled studies have indicated that patients with Crohn's disease may fare better with a high-protein, low-carbohydrate diet.[80] In my experience, there is no perfect diet for Crohn's disease, but my preference is to initiate treatment with the Specific Carbohydrate Diet (www.scdiet.com), which eliminates all cereal grains and disaccharides. It is essentially a Paleolithic diet with aged cheese sometimes permitted. One of its effects is to alter bacterial flora in the terminal ileum, an effect suggested by studies of patients with ileostomies. The caloric content of the diet can be enhanced by coconut oil, a source of medium-chain triglycerides; these triglycerides have been shown to exert an anti-inflammatory effect in inflammatory bowel disease, in contrast to other vegetable oils.

Supplementation with DHEA 200 mg/d, in men with inflammatory bowel disease and low serum DHEA, has reduced disease activities in a multiple case report,[81] so this was started, along with vitamin D3 (4000 IU/d) and zinc (25 mg/d). His abdominal pain, fever, and bleeding began diminishing within a week and were absent within a month, an unusually good response to diet therapy. His ESR decreased to 34 mm/h. Because of persistent diarrhea, a unique probiotic was added, *Saccharomyces boulardii*, a yeast with immune-modulating effects. It secretes a soluble anti-inflammatory factor and stimulates secretion of the anti-inflammatory cytokine interleukin-10.

Concluding Remarks

As we hope you have learned in this monograph, the gastrointestinal tract is a fulcrum through which a variety of systemic dysfunctions can occur. Thomas Sult, MD,[82] eloquently summarized its central importance in the *Textbook of Functional Medicine*:

> The GI system is the primary gateway by which the external environment interacts with the body. It serves as both portal and obstruction to the entry of substances into the human body, working continuously to distinguish beneficial from harmful influences, allowing entry to the former and denying entry to the latter....
>
> Most often, GI complaints are caused by multiple interdependent dysfunctions. Loss of digestion and absorption efficiency and integrity may lead to cascading, multisystem failure. Maldigestion can lead to symptoms of gas, bloating, diarrhea, pain, and/or constipation—that is, general irritability of the system. Gut irritability, left untreated, may lead to leaky gut and the development of food allergies, bacterial or yeast overgrowth, and the production of toxins. Toxins may accelerate the irritation and leakiness, resulting in toxic molecules entering the portal and then systemic circulation. This creates stress on systemic defenses, leading to immune, hormonal, or inflammatory imbalance....
>
> If there are a finite number of basic imbalances that affect the GI system, assessing for each and treating appropriately should have a profound impact on digestion and absorption. Indeed, clinically, this is the case, but the permutations are complex.... To help explain this complex interacting model, I use the analogy of the bike wheel. A typical wheel has 36 spokes. With even one spoke broken, the whole wheel will be thrown out of balance, making it likely that other spokes will break under the additional stress. In a short time, the wheel will be so out of true that it will no longer fit between the forks. At that point, the entire bike is useless. Similarly, our patients experience cascading, multisystem failure.

In this monograph, we have explored the vital components of gastrointestinal defense, what impairs their functionality, and what can be done to optimize them as part of an integrated approach to improving general physiological function. We have also explored how dysregulation of microflora, mucosal integrity, and the GALT can lead to systemic disease. In Chapters 3 and 4, we contrasted the conventional medical approach and the functional medicine approach to four conditions: irritable bowel syndrome, inflammatory bowel disease, rheumatoid arthritis, and fibromyalgia. And in this last chapter, we examined case studies and the effect of the 4R program for gut restoration and repair. This functional, *systems biology* framework allows clinicians to truly respond in a comprehensive manner to complex, chronic illnesses.

References

1. Jones DS, ed. *Textbook of Functional Medicine*. Gig Harbor, WA. The Institute for Functional Medicine; 2005.
2. Goldman L, Weinberg M, Weisberg M, et al. A computer-derived protocol to aid in the diagnosis of emergency room patients with acute chest pain. *N Engl J Med*. 1982;307:588-596.
3. Krumholz HM, Peterson ED, Ayanian JZ, et al. Report of the National Heart, Lung, and Blood Institute working group on outcomes research in cardiovascular disease. *Circulation*. 2005;111:3158-3166.
4. Holman H. Chronic disease--the need for a new clinical education. *JAMA*. 2004;292:1057-1059.
5. Levin B, Schmidt MA, Bland JS. Functional medicine in natural medicine. In: Pizzorno JE, Murray MT, eds. *Textbook of Natural Medicine*. Vol Volume 1. 2nd ed. St. Louis, MO: Churchill Livingston; 1999.
6. Osler W. Greek Medicine. In: Garrison FH, ed. *The Evolution of Modern Medicine*. New Haven, CT: Yale University Press; 1921:"Phaedrus replies: 'Hippocrates, the Asclepiad, says that the nature, even of the body, can only be understood as a whole' (Plato, I,311:III,270-Jowett, I,131,479)."
7. Vasquez A. *Integrative Rheumatology*. 2nd ed. Fort Worth, TX: Integrative and Biological Medicine Research and Consulting; 2007.
8. Seaman DR. The diet-induced proinflammatory state: a cause of chronic pain and other degenerative diseases? *J Manipulative Physiol Ther*. 2002;25:168-179.

9. Vasquez A. Reducing pain and inflammation naturally. Part 1: New insights into fatty acid biochemistry and the influence of diet. *Nutritional Perspectives*. 2004:5, 7-10, 12, 14.
10. Vasquez A. Reducing pain and inflammation naturally. Part 2: New insights into fatty acid supplementation and its effect on eicosanoid production and genetic expression. *Nutritional Perspectives*. 2005:5-16.
11. Vasquez A. Reducing pain and inflammation naturally. Part 3: Improving overall health while safely and effectively treating musculoskeletal pain. *Nutritional Perspectives*. 2005;28:34-38, 40-42.
12. Vasquez A. Reducing pain and inflammation naturally. Part 4: Nutritional and botanical inhibition of NF-kappaB, the major intracellular amplifier of the inflammatory cascade. A practical clinical strategy exemplifying anti-inflammatory nutrigenomics. *Nutritional Perspectives*. 2005:5-12.
13. Timms PM, Mannan N, Hitman GA, et al. Circulating MMP9, vitamin D and variation in the TIMP-1 response with VDR genotype: mechanisms for inflammatory damage in chronic disorders? *QJM*. 2002;95:787-796.
14. Al Faraj S, Al Mutairi K. Vitamin D deficiency and chronic low back pain in Saudi Arabia. *Spine*. 2003;28:177-179.
15. James MJ, Gibson RA, Cleland LG. Dietary polyunsaturated fatty acids and inflammatory mediator production. *Am J Clin Nutr*. 2000;71:343S-348S.
16. James MJ, Proudman SM, Cleland LG. Dietary n-3 fats as adjunctive therapy in a prototypic inflammatory disease: issues and obstacles for use in rheumatoid arthritis. *Prostaglandins Leukot Essent Fatty Acids*. 2003;68:399-405.
17. Mohanty P, Hamouda W, Garg R, Aljada A, Ghanim H, Dandona P. Glucose challenge stimulates reactive oxygen species (ROS) generation by leucocytes. *J Clin Endocrinol Metab*. 2000;85:2970-2973.
18. Mohanty P, Ghanim H, Hamouda W, Aljada A, Garg R, Dandona P. Both lipid and protein intakes stimulate increased generation of reactive oxygen species by polymorphonuclear leukocytes and mononuclear cells. *Am J Clin Nutr*. 2002;75:767-772.
19. Aljada A, Mohanty P, Ghanim H, et al. Increase in intranuclear nuclear factor kappaB and decrease in inhibitor kappaB in mononuclear cells after a mixed meal: evidence for a proinflammatory effect. *Am J Clin Nutr*. 2004;79:682-690.
20. Hitchon CA, El-Gabalawy HS. Oxidation in rheumatoid arthritis. *Arthritis Res Ther*. 2004;6:265-278.
21. Kurien BT, Hensley K, Bachmann M, Scofield RH. Oxidatively modified autoantigens in autoimmune diseases. *Free Radic Biol Med*. 2006;41:549-556.
22. Tak PP, Zvaifler NJ, Green DR, Firestein GS. Rheumatoid arthritis and p53: how oxidative stress might alter the course of inflammatory diseases. *Immunol Today*. 2000;21:78-82.
23. Park JH, Phothimat P, Oates CT, Hernanz-Schulman M, Olsen NJ. Use of P-31 magnetic resonance spectroscopy to detect metabolic abnormalities in muscles of patients with fibromyalgia. *Arthritis Rheum*. 1998;41:406-413.
24. Pieczenik SR, Neustadt J. Mitochondrial dysfunction and molecular pathways of disease. *Exp Mol Pathol*. 2007;83:84-92.
25. Grant EC. Food allergies and migraine. *Lancet*. 1979;1:966-969.
26. Millichap JG, Yee MM. The diet factor in pediatric and adolescent migraine. *Pediatr Neurol*. 2003;28:9-15.
27. Golding DN. Is there an allergic synovitis? *J R Soc Med*. 1990;83:312-314.
28. Hvatum M, Kanerud L, Hallgren R, Brandtzaeg P. The gut-joint axis: cross reactive food antibodies in rheumatoid arthritis. *Gut*. 2006;55:1240-1247.
29. van de Laar MA, Aalbers M, Bruins FG, van Dinther-Janssen AC, van der Korst JK, Meijer CJ. Food intolerance in rheumatoid arthritis. II. Clinical and histological aspects. *Ann Rheum Dis*. 1992;51:303-306.
30. Bourne JT, Kumar P, Huskisson EC, Mageed R, Unsworth DJ, Wojtulewski JA. Arthritis and coeliac disease. *Ann Rheum Dis*. 1985;44:592-598.
31. Corrigan FM, Wienburg CL, Shore RF, Daniel SE, Mann D. Organochlorine insecticides in substantia nigra in Parkinson's disease. *J Toxicol Environ Health A*. 2000;59:229-234.
32. Fleming L, Mann JB, Bean J, Briggle T, Sanchez-Ramos JR. Parkinson's disease and brain levels of organochlorine pesticides. *Ann Neurol*. 1994;36:100-103.
33. Fujiyoshi PT, Michalek JE, Matsumura F. Molecular epidemiologic evidence for diabetogenic effects of dioxin exposure in U.S. Air force veterans of the Vietnam war. *Environ Health Perspect*. 2006;114:1677-1683.
34. Lee DH, Lee IK, Jin SH, Steffes M, Jacobs DR, Jr. Association between serum concentrations of persistent organic pollutants and insulin resistance among nondiabetic adults: results from the National Health and Nutrition Examination Survey 1999-2002. *Diabetes Care*. 2007;30:622-628.
35. Lee DH, Lee IK, Song K, et al. A strong dose-response relation between serum concentrations of persistent organic pollutants and diabetes: results from the National Health and Examination Survey 1999-2002. *Diabetes Care*. 2006;29:1638-1644.
36. Remillard RB, Bunce NJ. Linking dioxins to diabetes: epidemiology and biologic plausibility. *Environ Health Perspect*. 2002;110:853-858.
37. Cheuk DK, Wong V. Attention-deficit hyperactivity disorder and blood mercury level: a case-control study in chinese children. *Neuropediatrics*. 2006;37:234-240.
38. Nigg JT, Knottnerus GM, Martel MM, et al. Low blood lead levels associated with clinically diagnosed attention-deficit/hyperactivity disorder and mediated by weak cognitive control. *Biol Psychiatry*. 2008;63:325-331.
39. Rauh VA, Garfinkel R, Perera FP, et al. Impact of prenatal chlorpyrifos exposure on neurodevelopment in the first 3 years of life among inner-city children. *Pediatrics*. 2006;118:e1845-1859.
40. Crinnion WJ. Results of a decade of naturopathic treatment for environmental illnesses: A review of clinical records. *Journal of Naturopathic Medicine*. 1997;7:21-27.
41. Crinnion WJ. Environmental medicine, part 2 - health effects of and protection from ubiquitous airborne solvent exposure. *Altern Med Rev*. 2000;5:133-143.
42. Crinnion WJ. Environmental medicine, part 4: pesticides - biologically persistent and ubiquitous toxins. *Altern Med Rev*. 2000;5:432-447.
43. Crinnion WJ. Environmental medicine, part one: the human burden of environmental toxins and their common health effects. *Altern Med Rev*. 2000;5:52-63.
44. Crinnion WJ. Environmental medicine, part three: long-term effects of chronic low-dose mercury exposure. *Altern Med Rev*. 2000;5:209-223.
45. Rea WJ, Pan Y, Johnson AR. Clearing of toxic volatile hydrocarbons from humans. *Bol Asoc Med P R*. 1991;83:321-324.
46. Bland JS, Barrager E, Reedy RG, Bland K. a Medical Food-Supplemented Detoxification Program in the Management of Chronic Health Problems. *Altern Ther Health Med*. 1995;1:62-71.
47. Minich DM, Bland JS. Acid-alkaline balance: role in chronic disease and detoxification. *Altern Ther Health Med*. 2007;13:62-65.
48. Vasquez A. Diabetes: Are toxins to blame? *Naturopathy Digest*. 2007;2.

49. Cecchini M, LoPresti V. Drug residues store in the body following cessation of use: impacts on neuroendocrine balance and behavior--use of the Hubbard sauna regimen to remove toxins and restore health. *Med Hypotheses.* 2007;68:868-879.
50. Kilburn KH, Warsaw RH, Shields MG. Neurobehavioral dysfunction in firemen exposed to polycholorinated biphenyls (PCBs): possible improvement after detoxification. *Arch Environ Health.* 1989;44:345-350.
51. Williams RJ. *Biochemical Individuality: The Basis for the Genetotrophic Concept.* Austin and London: University of Texas Press; 1956.
52. Pauling L. On the orthomolecular environment of the mind: Orthomolecular theory. In: Williams RJ, Kalita DK, eds. *A Physician's Handbook on Orthomolecular Medicine.* New Canaan, CT: Keats Publishing; 1977.
53. Pauling L, Robinson AB, Teranishi R, Cary P. Quantitative analysis of urine vapor and breath by gas-liquid partition chromatography. *Proc Natl Acad Sci U S A.* 1971;68:2374-2376.
54. Pauling L, Itano HA, et al. Sickle cell anemia a molecular disease. *Science.* 1949;110:543-548.
55. Evans JL, Maddux BA, Goldfine ID. The molecular basis for oxidative stress-induced insulin resistance. *Antioxid Redox Signal.* 2005;7:1040-1052.
56. Joseph JA, Denisova N, Fisher D, et al. Membrane and receptor modifications of oxidative stress vulnerability in aging. Nutritional considerations. *Ann N Y Acad Sci.* 1998;854:268-276.
57. Henrotte JG, Plouin PF, Levy-Leboyer C, et al. Blood and urinary magnesium, zinc, calcium, free fatty acids, and catecholamines in type A and type B subjects. *J Am Coll Nutr.* 1985;4:165-172.
58. Ingenbleek Y, Bernstein L. The stressful condition as a nutritionally dependent adaptive dichotomy. *Nutrition.* 1999;15:305-320.
59. Stephensen CB, Alvarez JO, Kohatsu J, Hardmeier R, Kennedy JI, Jr., Gammon RB, Jr. Vitamin A is excreted in the urine during acute infection. *Am J Clin Nutr.* 1994;60:388-392.
60. Imrich R. The role of neuroendocrine system in the pathogenesis of rheumatic diseases (minireview). *Endocr Regul.* 2002;36:95-106.
61. Orbach H, Shoenfeld Y. Hyperprolactinemia and autoimmune diseases. *Autoimmun Rev.* 2007;6:537-542.
62. Panush RS, Wallace DJ, Dorff RE, Engleman EP. Retraction of the suggestion to use the term "Reiter's syndrome" sixty-five years later: the legacy of Reiter, a war criminal, should not be eponymic honor but rather condemnation. *Arthritis Rheum.* 2007;56:693-694.
63. Collins SM. Stress and the Gastrointestinal Tract IV. Modulation of intestinal inflammation by stress: basic mechanisms and clinical relevance. *Am J Physiol Gastrointest Liver Physiol.* 2001;280:G315-318.
64. Farhadi A, Fields JZ, Keshavarzian A. Mucosal mast cells are pivotal elements in inflammatory bowel disease that connect the dots: stress, intestinal hyperpermeability and inflammation. *World J Gastroenterol.* 2007;13:3027-3030.
65. Hart A, Kamm MA. Review article: mechanisms of initiation and perpetuation of gut inflammation by stress. *Aliment Pharmacol Ther.* 2002;16:2017-2028.
66. Rashid T, Ebringer A. Ankylosing spondylitis is linked to Klebsiella-the evidence. *Clin Rheumatol.* 2007;26:858-864.
67. Samarkos M, Vaiopoulos G. The role of infections in the pathogenesis of autoimmune diseases. *Curr Drug Targets Inflamm Allergy.* 2005;4:99-103.
68. Tlaskalova-Hogenova H, Stepankova R, Hudcovic T, et al. Commensal bacteria (normal microflora), mucosal immunity and chronic inflammatory and autoimmune diseases. *Immunol Lett.* 2004;93:97-108.
69. Yang PC, Jury J, Soderholm JD, Sherman PM, McKay DM, Perdue MH. Chronic psychological stress in rats induces intestinal sensitization to luminal antigens. *Am J Pathol.* 2006;168:104-114; quiz 363.
70. Alverdy J, Holbrook C, Rocha F, et al. Gut-derived sepsis occurs when the right pathogen with the right virulence genes meets the right host: evidence for in vivo virulence expression in Pseudomonas aeruginosa. *Ann Surg.* 2000;232:480-489.
71. Wu L, Holbrook C, Zaborina O, et al. Pseudomonas aeruginosa expresses a lethal virulence determinant, the PA-I lectin/adhesin, in the intestinal tract of a stressed host: the role of epithelia cell contact and molecules of the Quorum Sensing Signaling System. *Ann Surg.* 2003;238:754-764.
72. Knowler WC, Barrett-Connor E, Fowler SE, et al. Reduction in the incidence of type 2 diabetes with lifestyle intervention or metformin. *N Engl J Med.* 2002;346:393-403.
73. Tuomilehto J, Lindstrom J. The major diabetes prevention trials. *Curr Diab Rep.* 2003;3:115-122.
74. Grundy SM. N-3 fatty acids: priority for post-myocardial infarction clinical trials. *Circulation.* 2003;107:1834-1836.
75. Burr ML, Fehily AM, Gilbert JF, et al. Effects of changes in fat, fish, and fibre intakes on death and myocardial reinfarction: diet and reinfarction trial (DART). *Lancet.* 1989;2:757-761.
76. de Lorgeril M, Renaud S, Mamelle N, et al. Mediterranean alpha-linolenic acid-rich diet in secondary prevention of coronary heart disease. *Lancet.* 1994;343:1454-1459.
77. Sudak N, Shapiro V. Identifying practical interventions that help to normalize multiple symptoms. In: Jones DS, ed. *Textbook of Functional Medicine.* Gig Harbor, WA: The Institute for Functional Medicine; 2005:709-712.
78. Galland L. *The Fat Resistance Diet.* New York, NY: Broadway Books; 2005.
79. Basivireddy J, Jacob M, Balasubramanian KA. Oral glutamine attenuates indomethacin-induced small intestinal damage. *Clin Sci (Lond).* 2004;107:281-289.
80. Lorenz-Meyer H, Bauer P, Nicolay C, et al. Omega-3 fatty acids and low carbohydrate diet for maintenance of remission in Crohn's disease. A randomized controlled multicenter trial. Study Group Members (German Crohn's Disease Study Group). *Scand J Gastroenterol.* 1996;31:778-785.
81. Andus T, Klebl F, Rogler G, Bregenzer N, Scholmerich J, Straub RH. Patients with refractory Crohn's disease or ulcerative colitis respond to dehydroepiandrosterone: a pilot study. *Aliment Pharmacol Ther.* 2003;17:409-414.
82. Sult T. Digestion and absorption. In: Jones DS, ed. *Textbook of Functional Medicine.* Gig Harbor, WA: The Institute for Functional Medicine; 2005:435-444.

Appendix

The 4R Program[i]

Gastrointestinal complaints are among the leading reasons patients seek out healthcare practitioners. In the United States, more than 70 million patients suffer some form of gastrointestinal disorder, which can range from mild discomfort to life-threatening disease. Frequently diagnosed gastrointestinal-related conditions include gastro-esophageal reflux disease, gastritis, peptic ulcer, cholecystitis, diverticulitis, and inflammatory bowel disease. Even more common is the so-called "functional" disorder of irritable bowel syndrome.[1,2] Many of the most common gastrointestinal disorders are found with greater frequency in people over 60 years of age and, therefore, are on the rise due to the aging of our population.[3]

While conditions localized to the gastrointestinal tract make for an extensive list, gastrointestinal dysfunction has also been linked to a number of other non-localized systemic conditions. This connection is likely related to a breech in the intestinal barrier, and is often referred to as "leaky gut." Increased intestinal permeability can lead to many systemic inflammatory and immune-related symptoms. It has been implicated in such unrelated conditions as rheumatoid arthritis, ankylosing spondylitis, eczema, non-alcoholic fatty liver disease, and chronic urticaria.[4,5,6,7,8,9,10,11] Thus, the normal integrity of the gastrointestinal tract may be compromised, resulting in distant systemic complaints, even in the absence of overt gastrointestinal symptomatology.

The ability of the body to maintain healthy gastrointestinal function, and to heal the gastrointestinal barrier when its integrity is breached, is integral to protection from many diseases and disorders. However, maintenance of healthy gastrointestinal function is not a simple task, and understanding how to evaluate and therapeutically support gastrointestinal function can be a difficult undertaking in a busy practice. For that reason, this appendix provides an in-depth discussion of a well-established functional medicine approach to treating gastrointestinal dysfunction. This method for identifying clinical assessments and interventions that focus on normalizing and optimizing gastrointestinal function has been referred to as the "4R" program, in reference to its four basic clinical steps: remove, replace, reinoculate, and repair. It is designed to provide a focus for evaluation of the status of gastrointestinal function, with interventions targeted to appropriate nutritional, digestive, probiotic/prebiotic, and antimicrobial therapy. The specific application of the program depends on the nature and course of the patient's condition and should be individualized for maximum effectiveness.

[i] The Appendix was adapted from Lukaczer D. The "4R" Program." In: Jones DS, ed. *Textbook of Functional Medicine*. Gig Harbor, WA: The Institute for Functional Medicine; 2005.

The 4R Model

Often in conventional medicine, the clinician asks only how to suppress a particular symptom in a patient. The 4R model asks four primary questions in a patient with gastrointestinal-related complaints, or complaints whose origins may stem from a breach of gastrointestinal mucosal integrity:

1. What may need to be *removed* to support healthy gastrointestinal function? The clinician may need to assess the presence/activity of pathogenic or potentially pathogenic yeast, bacteria, or protozoa in the intestinal tract, or foods and additives that result in allergic or intolerant responses.
2. What may need to be *replaced* to support healthy gastrointestinal function? Digestive enzymes, bile salts, or stomach acid secretions should be considered.
3. What may be needed to support and/or reestablish a healthy balance of microflora? This step may include *reinoculation* with probiotic and/or prebiotics.
4. What may be needed to support regeneration and *repair* of a healthy mucosal layer? A variety of specific nutrients and phytonutrients are available for this purpose.

Remove

The "remove" aspect of this model focuses on eliminating pathogenic bacteria, viruses, fungi, parasites, and other environmentally-derived toxic substances from the gastrointestinal tract. Foods themselves may be the most important offending agents. Over the course of a lifetime, the gastrointestinal tract processes many tons of food, representing the largest antigenic load confronting the human immune system.[12] (Experts vary on the tonnage, but figures range from 30 to 60 tons of food consumed in the lifetime of the average well-nourished adult.[13]) During digestion, proteins and large peptides are broken down into amino acids or small peptides within the intestinal lumen, which removes or decreases their antigenic potential. In a healthy intestinal tract, more than 98% of ingested food antigens are blocked from entering circulation by a host of gastrointestinal barrier functions (described earlier in this chapter). In a compromised environment with increased intestinal permeability, significantly more antigens may penetrate to the systemic circulation. These protein fragments, recognized as foreign molecules, stimulate an immune response. In genetically susceptible individuals, autoimmune reactions may therefore result from this increased antigenic load.

Not every adverse response to food qualifies as an immunologically-mediated food allergy. By definition, an immune response only occurs when an antigen/antibody reaction has taken place. Therefore, if a person does not have antibodies against a specific food antigen, he or she cannot have an allergic reaction to that food. However, patients do respond in non-immunological ways. A simple example is a lactase insufficiency, which underlies lactose intolerance, and would not be considered an allergic reaction. Many food reactions fall into this category.

Some controversy exists with respect to the actual definition of food allergy. Some definitions describe a true food allergy as only an IgE-mediated response, which is also called a type 1 hypersensitivity, whereas a substance that elicits antibodies of any other class is termed antigenic. However, it is becoming clear that not all symptoms of allergic responses can be ascribed to IgE-mediated mechanisms.[14] Many allergic responses appear to involve some form of prolonged or delayed reactions to allergens.[15] IgG antibodies have been implicated as a possible etiological factor in conditions such as atopic dermatitis, asthma and IBS.[16,17,18] Therefore, there appears to be some evidence for a role of both IgE and IgG antibodies in the provocation of both immediate and delayed reactions to food allergens.

Food allergies have been suggested as the cause of a variety of symptoms. Clinical studies suggest that 8% of U.S. children younger than six years have evidence of food intolerance, and 2 to 4% of those experience reproducible allergic reactions to foods, most often eggs, milk, peanuts, soy, fish, and wheat.[19,20] Surveys suggest that 1 to 2% of adult Americans are sensitive to foods, most commonly nuts, peanuts, fish, and shellfish.[21,22,23] Because delayed food

Table 1—Symptoms and Diseases that may be Associated with Food Allergy

System	Symptoms/Disease
Gastrointestinal	Canker sores, celiac disease, chronic diarrhea, stomach ulcers, duodenal ulcers, recurrent mouth ulcers, indigestion, nausea, vomiting, diarrhea, constipation, gas, gastritis, irritable bowel syndrome, malabsorption, ulcerative colitis, Crohn's disease, colic (babies)
Genitourinary	Bed wetting, chronic bladder infections, nephrotic syndrome, frequent urination
HEENT	Serous otitis media, migraine headaches
Mental/Emotional	Attention deficit disorder, depression, anxiety, memory loss, epileptic seizures, schizophrenia
Musculoskeletal	Joint pain, myalgias, rheumatoid arthritis
Respiratory	Asthma, chronic or allergic sinusitis, constant runny or congested nose, nasal polyps
Cardiovascular	Irregular heart rhythm, vasculitis, inflammation of the veins producing purpura, spontaneous bruising, urticaria, edema
Skin	Eczema, psoriasis, urticaria, red itchy eyes, itchy skin

reactions are often difficult to diagnose, these figures likely under-represent the extent of food allergy in the population. Table 1 lists some common symptoms and diseases that have been associated with food allergies.

The underlying mechanisms that elicit food-intolerant or allergic responses are complex and controversial, and a variety of assessment techniques for food allergy have been developed. Unfortunately, none are completely adequate, and it appears that the most cost-effective and accurate avenue to determine food allergy is the elimination or oligoantigenic diet, containing only those foods known to pose little risk of an allergic or intolerant reaction. Several studies have shown an association between food allergy and a variety of diseases and symptoms, with avoidance of the suspected foods leading to substantial improvement in clinical symptoms. Therefore, oligoantigenic diets are typically part of a "remove" protocol.[24,25] If a clinician or patient wants to confirm food sensitivity, the potentially offending food can be reintroduced and symptoms monitored.

Equally important in assessment of antigenic stimuli is the myriad array of organisms that reside in or invade the gastrointestinal system. All too often, gut flora assessment is overlooked as a significant source of information concerning systemic or even local health problems. Recognition that intestinal flora could have a major impact on health and disease was first popularized by the Russian scientist Eli Metchnikoff at the turn of the 20th century. Metchnikoff put forth the idea of "dysbiosis," which he defined as a state of living with intestinal flora that may have harmful or detrimental effects. That idea is now receiving significant scientific validation. The indigenous flora was once thought to be relatively benign. It seems clear that the subject is far more complicated than previously believed.

The number of bacteria in the large bowel alone is greater than 100 billion, which is more than the total number of cells in the human body. These bacteria constitute a powerful chemical factory and can have important effects on human physiology depending upon their activities. Intestinal bacteria produce toxins and antitoxins, alter chemical composition of foods and drugs, produce and degrade vitamins, produce short-chain fatty acids (SCFAs) from fiber, degrade dietary toxins, and inhibit the growth of certain pathogens. Bacterial by-products can inactivate brush border and pancreatic enzymes, deconjugate bile salts, and hydrolyze bile acids. Problems from a dysbiotic condition often relate to the prolific activity of an altered intestinal microflora. Additionally, through the process of microbial translocation, defined as the passage of both viable and nonviable microbes and microbial products (endotoxins) across an anatomically intact intestinal barrier, gut-derived products may play a role in increasing the systemic immune inflammatory response.[26] There is evidence that microflora share antigenic determinants with normal tissue and produce cross-reactive antibodies.[27,28] Bacterial lipopolysaccharides found in the cell walls of gram-negative bacteria have been shown to initiate immune responses and elevate proinflammatory cytokines.[29] For example, inflammatory diseases of the bowel (such as Crohn's and ulcerative colitis), rheumatoid arthritis, and other spondyloarthropathies have been linked to indigenous flora of the gut.[28,30,3132,33]

Yeast is another example of indigenous flora that may have detrimental consequences. There is evidence that, in certain individuals, intestinal yeast may result in a wide variety of symptomatology.[34,35] Although still controversial, the "yeast syndrome" further supports the hypothesis that intestinal organisms can cause or exacerbate systemic or local disease.

The distinction between what is and what is not a pathogen becomes increasingly muddled when one looks at organisms that are clearly not indigenous. Certain parasites, yeasts, and bacteria are traditionally associated with local and systemic consequences. Examples are pathogenic strains of *Salmonella*, *Giardia*, *Shigella*, and *Campylobacter*. However, it does not appear that what has been traditionally described as a pathogen always elicits the same response. Diverse pathogens have been termed weak or strong, and pathogenicity may be determined in part by host immunological competence.[36] An example is the protozoa *Blastocystis hominis*. Experts disagree sharply on its pathogenicity. In certain studies, it has been associated with colitis, diarrhea, and other gastrointestinal complaints.[37,38,39,40] Other studies show it to be equally present in asymptomatic and symptomatic individuals, suggesting that it may not always be pathogenic.[41] Weak pathogens may cause disease in some people some of the time. Host resistance and virulence factors are important. Weakly pathogenic strains of *Salmonella*, *Giardia*, and yeast may be other examples of this theme.[42]

Pathogens can take up colonization anywhere in the gastrointestinal mucosa, and cell wall components of bacteria, yeasts, and protozoa can be absorbed, which may cause systemic symptoms that are difficult to pinpoint to the pathogen directly. Laboratory tests evaluating microbiology, parasites, and presence of serum antibodies to pathogens are often useful to verify unwanted microbial organisms in the gastrointestinal tract and monitor response to treatment.

Thus, bacteria, yeasts, and parasites may cause symptoms locally as well as systemically. Food proteins, gut bacterial breakdown products, and environmental toxins can and do reach the systemic circulation. Therefore, removal of offending antigens becomes key to a gastrointestinal restoration program.

Replace

The second clinical step in the 4R program, "replace," replenishes enzymes and other digestive factors which may be lacking or limited. Enzymes that may at times need to be replaced include proteases, lipases, cellulases, and saccharidases, which are normally secreted by cells lining the intestine or directly by the pancreas. Other digestive factors that may require replenishment include hydrochloric acid, pepsin, and intrinsic factor, normally secreted by cells in the stomach wall, and bile, synthesized by hepatocytes.

A key ingredient in replacement therapies is hydrochloric acid. Low stomach acidity can result in a variety of symptoms and digestive problems. It is particularly common among individuals older than 60. Reduced hydrochloric acid may impair the absorption of nutrients such as vitamin B6, folic acid, calcium, and iron and may also predispose an individual to increased intestinal infections. As hydrochloric acid production depends on zinc, decreased levels may indicate a zinc deficiency as well.[43]

The small intestine acts as the principal site of digestion and absorption. As mentioned, intact proteins and other large molecules can cross the intestinal lining, even in healthy individuals, to a certain extent.[44,45] Therapies that involve digestive enzyme supplementation enhance the breakdown of these particles and therefore help to exclude them from crossing that barrier intact. A variety of health conditions, including eczema and steatorrhea, may be ameliorated by enzyme therapy. For example, studies have shown that the digestive enzyme lipase, critical in fat digestion, can be supplemented to relieve problems of fat malabsorption.[46,47,48] Similarly, many people suffer from undiagnosed lactose intolerance. The digestive enzyme, lactase, has also been used successfully in individuals with the inability to digest lactose.[49]

Food allergies are another area where digestive enzymes may be helpful. Food allergies can be caused by several factors, including the increased supply of intact, poorly digested protein fragments that leak across the gut wall into the systemic circulation. By increasing digestion of dietary protein, protease enzymes decrease the supply of intact proteins available to leak into the bloodstream. Digestive protease enzymes taken orally may also help to digest dietary proteins that are encountered in the bloodstream. Table 2 provides some general information on the indications and approaches to the use of HCl and digestive enzymes. Laboratory tests such as gastric analyses, fat absorption tests, and stool analyses may be useful tools to verify the need to replace enzymes and other digestive factors.

Reinoculate

"Reinoculate" is the third step in the 4R gastrointestinal support program. Reinoculate refers to the reintroduction of desirable bacteria, or "probiotics," into the intestine to reestablish microflora balance. Bacterial balance in the intestine is critical for proper intestinal permeability. Over 400 different species of microorganisms reside in the human gastrointestinal tract and the overall balance of these organisms can profoundly influence gut ecology and health.

Probiotics serve a variety of functions in the gastrointestinal tract. Perhaps the most important function of probiotics is antagonistic activity toward pathogens, which they perform in a variety of complementary ways. First, probiotics assist in colonization resistance—the ability of normal flora to protect against the unwanted establishment of pathogens. Second, probiotics may produce various antimicrobial substances. For instance, *Lactobacillus casei GG* has been shown to produce substances inhibitory toward a broad spectrum of gram-positive and gram-negative pathogens.[50] Competition for nutrients is a third mechanism. By competing for available nutrient substrate, beneficial bacteria can inhibit the growth of other less favorable flora. Competitive inhibition for bacterial adhesion sites is a fourth mechanism of probiotics. For instance, *Lactobacillus acidophilus* inhibits the adhesion of several enteric pathogens to human intestinal cells.[51] A final mechanism involves systemic host response. For instance, *L. casei GG*, administered orally to subjects with Crohn's disease, promoted a secretory IgA (sIgA) response.[52] These varied actions may decrease the likelihood that pathogens will develop resistance against probiotic agents. Thus, probiotics may be viewed as a vehicle to neutralize or inhibit pathogen activities, or increase or stimulate host immune stimulant activities to the intestinal tract, or both.[53]

A variety of supplemental sources may be considered helpful in reinoculation. These include cultured and fermented foods containing live bacteria, refrigerated liquid supplements containing live bacteria, or freeze-dried bac-

Table 2 — Using Digestive Enzymes and Hydrochloric Acid

Possible Symptoms of Low Stomach Acid	Taking HCl Supplements	Using Digestive Enzymes
• Bloating, belching, burning, and flatulence immediately after meals • Dilated blood vessels in the nose or cheeks (Rosacea) • Excess gas in the upper intestine • Indigestion, diarrhea, or constipation • Iron deficiency • Multiple food allergies • Nausea after taking supplements • Peeling or cracking fingernails • Rectal itching • Sense of "fullness" after eating • Undigested food in the stool	• Find supplements with at least 600 mg of betaine HCl per tablet or capsule. • Start with one right at the beginning of a meal or immediately after beginning to eat. • At every meal after that, use one more pill. • Continue until 5 tablets/capsules are consumed with each meal, or until warmth occurs in the stomach, whichever occurs first. • The warm feeling indicates too many were consumed, so cut back by one pill at the next meal. • Smaller meals need fewer pills, larger meals more. • Those who need 5 or so capsules should spread them throughout the meal. • After a while, and after repairing the digestive system, patients may produce their own HCl and need fewer capsules. The "warmth" will be present with fewer capsules. Just cut down the dose at that point.	Effective enzymes are available from both animal and plant sources; some are also available by prescription. Use 2–3 just before or at the beginning of a meal. They are generally well tolerated and without side effects. Look for a formula containing at least: • Protease 100,000 USP units • Lipase 20,000 USP units • Amylase 100,000 USP units Vegetarians can take a mixed plant-based form of digestive enzymes. Use 2–3 just before or at the beginning of a meal. Some of these are grown from Aspergillus fungus, so be careful if the patient has mold or yeast sensitivities. Others are derived from pineapple (bromelain) and papaya. Look for a formula with about 500 mg of enzymes per tablet or capsule and containing: • Amylase 100,000 USP units • Protease 100,000 USP units • Lipase 10,000 USP units • Lactase 1600 Lace Digestive bitters may also be tried. Swedish bitters or other aperitifs stimulate digestive function. Herbal bitters including gentian (most common) and artichoke, cardamom, fennel, ginger, and dandelion are also available in more concentrated forms that can be added to water.

teria packaged in powder, tablet, or capsule form. Frequently supplemented species include *Lactobacillus acidophilus, Lactobacillus bulgaricus, Lactobacillus thermophilus, Lactobacillus sporogenes, Lactobacillus casei GG, Lactobacillus NCFM, Saccharomyces boulardii, Bifidobacterium bifidus, Bifidobacterium longum,* and *Bifidobacterium breve.*

In addition to directly reintroducing bacteria, the reinoculate step may also involve indirectly bolstering the healthy microflora with prebiotics, which selectively promote beneficial synergistic flora without simultaneously supporting pathogenic bacterial growth. When prebiotics are included in the diet, increased levels of fecal fermentation and intraluminal concentrations of SCFAs, such as propionate, acetate, and butyrate, are produced from fermentation of the fibers by the colonic microflora. SCFAs are thought to supply up to 70% of the energy used by colonic epithelial cells; therefore, prebiotics support improved intestinal integrity and promote intestinal mucosal cell regeneration.[54] Prebiotics include fructans, inulin and fructooligosaccharides, arabinogalactans and some soy fibers.[54,55,56,57] The incorporation of soluble fiber, another important nutrient substrate for probiotics, may also help in the reinoculation process.

Repair

The fourth and final step in a 4R approach is "repair." Repair refers to providing nutritional support for regeneration and healing of the gastrointestinal mucosa. Part of the support for healing comes from removing insults that continually re-injure or irritate the mucosa, and from promoting healthy microflora. The repair phase of gastrointestinal restoration benefits from all of the clinical approaches discussed so far.

The gastrointestinal mucosal cells represent the largest mass (in normal individuals) of rapidly proliferating cells. Repair is necessary whenever there has been a loss of integrity of the gastrointestinal mucosal structure, function, or both. This loss may be the result of chronic nutritional insufficiency, food allergen and xenobiotic exposure, dysbiosis, pathological intestinal infection, chronic inflammation as in ulcerative colitis, or other less common gastrointestinal diseases. Assessment of individual need may include a dietary history, nutritional analysis, and any other investigative techniques that reveal the presence of dysfunction, disease, or nutritional insufficiencies.

Once the need for repair has been determined, remediation of any process that resulted in intestinal damage must be done first; second, direct nutritional support of the intestinal cells should be provided through foods or supplements critical to intestinal wall structure and function. Nutrients that play pivotal roles in gastrointestinal mucosal cell differentiation, growth, functioning, and repair include glutamine, essential fatty acids, zinc and pantothenic acid. For instance, dietary deficiency of glutamine is associated with atrophy and degenerative changes in the small intestine following intestinal injury, infection, stress, surgery, and radiation.[58,59,60] Fish oils, which contain eicosapentaenoic acid and docosahexaenoic acid, have also been shown to ameliorate mucosal injury and attenuate inflammatory conditions of the gut in animal studies.[61,62,63,64] Research has shown that supplementation with pantothenic acid is important to support the normal healing process.[65] It has also been found that pantothenic acid is concentrated in gut mucosa and may be important for stimulating the regeneration of the gastrointestinal mucosa in individuals who have chronic ulcerative or granulomatous colitis.[66] Many individuals with inflammatory bowel disease have zinc deficiencies.[67,68,69,70]

Summary

The *Remove, Replace, Reinoculate, Repair* clinical approach is a conceptual program, meant to outline the points to consider when clinically evaluating and applying therapies to a patient with underlying gastrointestinal dysfunction. While this overall concept describes a basic approach, its use is individualized to the needs of each patient, based on his or her unique clinical condition and nutrient needs. The different steps in this gut restoration program can be applied together, in a unified therapy, or sequentially, beginning with *Remove*. When considered together, the steps of the 4R gastrointestinal support program may address a variety of clinical conditions. Proper assessment of gastrointestinal function and intervention in areas of dysfunction, imbalance, or impairment may have profound effects at the local as well as systemic level.

References

1. Horwitz BJ, Fisher RS. The irritable bowel syndrome. *N Engl J Med.* 2001;344:1846-1850.
2. Mayer EA. Emerging disease model for functional gastrointestinal disorders. *Am J Med.* 1999;107(5A):12S-19S.
3. Camilleri M, Lee JS, Viramontes B, Bharucha AE, Tangalos EG. Insights into the pathophysiology and mechanisms of constipation, irritable bowel syndrome, and diverticulosis in older people. *J Am Geriatr Soc.* 2000;48:1142-2250.
4. Mielants H, De Vos M, Goemaere S, et al. Intestinal mucosal permeability in inflammatory rheumatic diseases, part 2. *J Rheumatol.* 1991;18:394-400.
5. Andre C, Andre F, Colin L. Effect of allergen ingestion challenge with and without cromoglycate cover on intestinal permeability in atopic dermatitis, urticaria and other symptoms of food allergy. *Allergy.* 1989;44(Suppl 9):47-51.
6. Smith MD, Gibson RA, Brooks PM. Abnormal bowel permeability in ankylosing spondylitis and rheumatoid arthritis. *J Rheumatol.* 1985;12:299-305.
7. Isolauri E, Juntunen M, Wiren S, Vuorinen P, Koivula T. Intestinal permeability changes in acute gastroenteritis: effects of clinical factors and nutritional management. *J Pediatr Gastroenterol Nutr.* 1989;8:466-473.

8. Munkholm P, Langholz E, Hollander D, et al. Intestinal permeability in patients with Crohn's disease and ulcerative colitis and their first degree relatives. *Gut.* 1994;35:68-72.
9. Olaison G, Sjodahl R, Tagesson D. Abnormal intestinal permeability in Crohn's disease. A possible pathogenic factor. *Scand J Gastroenterol.* 1990;25:321-328.
10. Hollander D. Intestinal permeability, leaky gut, and intestinal disorders. *Curr Gastroenterol Rep.* 1999;1:410-416.
11. DeMeo MT, Mutlu EA, Keshavarzian A, Tobin MC. Intestinal permeation and gastrointestinal disease. *J Clin Gastroenterol.* 2002;34:385-396.
12. Sampson HA, Anderson JA. Summary and recommendations: Classification of gastrointestinal manifestations due to immunologic reactions to foods in infants and young children. *J Pediatr Gastroenterol Nutr.* 2000;(Suppl 30):S87-94.
13. Brandtzaeg PE. Current understanding of gastrointestinal immunoregulation and its relation to food allergy. *Ann N Y Acad Sci.* 2002;964:13-45.
14. Carini C, Brostoff J, Wraith DG. IgE complexes in food allergy. *Ann Allergy.* 1987;59:110-117.
15. Halpern GM, Scott JR. Non-IgE antibody mediated mechanisms in food allergy. *Ann Allergy.* 1987;58:14-27.
16. el Rafei A, Peters SM, Harris N, Bellanti JA. Diagnostic value of IgG4 measurements in patients with food allergy. *Ann Allergy.* 1989;62:94-99.
17. Atkinson W, Sheldon TA, Shaath N, Whorwell PJ. Food elimination based on IgG antibodies in irritable bowel syndrome: a randomised controlled trial. *Gut.* 2004;53:1459-1464.
18. Zar S, Kumar D, Benson MJ. Food hypersensitivity and irritable bowel syndrome. *Aliment Pharmacol Ther.* 2001;15:439-449.
19. Sampson HA. Clinical manifestations of adverse food reactions. *Pediatr Allergy Immunol.* 1995;6(Suppl 8):29-37.
20. Burks A, Sampson HA. Diagnostic approaches to the patient with suspected food allergies. *J Pediatr.* 1992;121(5 Pt 2):S64-71.
21. Carini C, Brostoff J, Wraith DG. IgE complexes in food allergy. *Ann Allergy.* 1987;59:110-117.
22. Halpern GM, Scott JR. Non-IgE antibody mediated mechanisms in food allergy. *Ann Allergy.* 1987;58:14-27.
23. Sampson HA. Clinical manifestations of adverse food reactions. *Pediatr Allergy Immunol.* 1995;6(Suppl 8):29-37.
24. Sicherer SH. Manifestations of food allergy: evaluation and management. *Am Fam Physician.* 1999;5:415-424, 429-430.
25. Sicherer SH, Sampson HA. Food hypersensitivity and atopic dermatitis: pathophysiology, epidemiology, diagnosis, and management. *J Allergy Clin Immunol.* 1999;104(3 Pt 2):S114-122.
26. Alexander JW, Boyce ST, Babcock GF, et al. The process of microbial translocation. *Ann Surg.* 1990;212:496-510.
27. Ebringer A, Khalafpour S, Wilson C. Rheumatoid arthritis and Proteus: a possible aetiological association. *Rheumatol Int.* 1989;9(3-5):223-328.
28. Rashid T, Leirisalo-Repo M, Tani Y, et al. Antibacterial and antipeptide antibodies in Japanese and Finnish patients with rheumatoid arthritis. *Clin Rheumatol.* 2004;23:134-141.
29. Pledger JV, Pearson AD, Craft AW, Laker MF, Eastham EJ. Intestinal permeability during chemotherapy for childhood tumours. *Eur J Pediatr.* 1988;147:123-127.
30. Pirzer U, Schonhaar A, Fleischer B, Hermann E, Meyer zum Büschenfelde KH. Reactivity of infiltrating T lymphocytes with microbial antigens in Crohn's disease. *Lancet.* 1991; 338(8777):1238-1239.
31. Falgarone G, Jaen O, Boissier MC. Role for innate immunity in rheumatoid arthritis. *Joint Bone Spine.* 2005;72:17-25.
32. Mills JA. Do bacteria cause chronic polyarthritis? *N Engl J Med.* 1989;320.245-246.
33. Gautam V, Sehgal R, Paramjeet SG, Arora DR. Detection of anti-Proteus antibodies in sera of patients with rheumatoid arthritis. *Indian J Pathol Microbiol.* 2003;46.137-141.
34. Kane JG, Chretien JH, Garagusi VF. Diarrhoea caused by Candida. *Lancet.* 1976;1(7955):335-336.
35. Bolivar RBG. Candidiasis of the gastrointestinal tract. In: *Candidiasis*, Bodey GP, Fainstein V, eds. New York, NY: Raven Press: 181-201.
36. Lee M. Parasites, yeasts and bacteria in health and disease. *J Adv Med.* 1995;8:121-229.
37. Tungtrongchitr A, Manatsathit S, Kositchaiwat C, et al. Blastocystic hominis infection in irritable bowel syndrome patients. *Southeast Asian J Trop Med Public Health.* 2004;35:705-710.
38. Carrascosa M, Martinez J, Perez-Castrillon JL. Hemorrhagic proctosigmoiditis and Blastocystis hominis infection. *Ann Int Med.* 1996:124:278-279.
39. Yarze JC. Hemorrhagic proctosigmoiditis and Blastocystis hominis. *Ann Int Med.* 2996;125:860-861.
40. Yakoob J, Jafri W, Jafri N, et al. Irritable bowel syndrome: in search of an etiology: role of Blastocystis hominis. *Am J Trop Med Hyg.* 2004;70:383-385.
41. Udkow MP, Markell EK. Blastocystis hominis: prevalence in asymptomatic versus symptomatic hosts. *J Infect Dis.* 1993;168:242-244.
42. Lee M. Parasites, yeasts and bacteria in health and disease. *J Adv Med.* 1995;8:121-129.
43. Cho CH. Zinc: absorption and role in gastrointestinal metabolism and disorders. *Dig Dis.* 1991;9:49-60.
44. Salamat-Miller N, Johnston TP. Current strategies used to enhance the paracellular transport of therapeutic polypeptides across the intestinal epithelium. Int J Pharm. 2005;294(1-2):201-216.
45. Gardner ML. Gastrointestinal absorption of intact proteins. Annu Rev Nutr. 1988;8:329-350.
46. Lu C-L, Chen C-Y, Luo J-C, et al. Impaired gastric myoelectricity in patients with chronic pancreatitis: role of maldigestion. *World J Gastroenterol.* 2005;11:372-376.
47. Griffin SM, Alderson D, Farndon JR. Acid resistant lipase as replacement therapy in chronic pancreatic exocrine insufficiency: a study in dogs. *Gut.* 1989;30:1012-1015.
48. Schneider MU, Knoll-Ruzicka ML, Domschke S, Heptner G, Domschke W. Pancreatic enzyme replacement therapy: comparative effects of conventional and enteric-coated microspheric pancreatin and acid-stable fungal enzyme preparations on steatorrhoea in chronic pancreatitis. *Hepatogastroenterology.* 1985;32:97-102.
49. Barillas C, Solomons NW. Effective reduction of lactose maldigestion in preschool children by direct addition of beta-galactosidases to milk at mealtime. *Pediatrics.* 1987;79:766-772.
50. Silva M, Jacobus NV, Deneke C, Gorbach SL. Antimicrobial substance from a human Lactobacillus strain. *Antimicrob Agents Chemother.* 1987;31:1231-1233.
51. Bernet MF, Brassart D, Neeser JR, Servin AL. Lactobacillus acidophilus LA 1 binds to cultured human intestinal cell lines and inhibits cell attachment and cell invasion by enterovirulent bacteria. *Gut.* 1994;35:483-489.
52. Malin M, Suomalainen H, Saxelin M, Isolauri E. Promotion of IgA immune response in patients with Crohn's disease by oral bacteriotherapy with Lactobacillus GG. *Ann Nutr Metab.* 1996;40:137-145.
53. Elmer GW, Surawicz CM, McFarland LV. Biotherapeutic agents. A neglected modality for the treatment and prevention of selected intestinal and vaginal infections. *JAMA.* 1996;275:870-876.

54. Gibson GR, Roberfroid MB. Dietary modulation of the human colonic microbiota: introducing the concept of prebiotics. *J Nutr.* 1995;125:1401-1412.
55. Roberfroid MB. Chicory fructooligosaccharides and the gastrointestinal tract. *Nutrition.* 2000;16(7-8):677-679.
56. Robinson RR, Feirtag J, Slavin JL. Effects of dietary arabinogalactan on gastrointestinal and blood parameters in healthy human subjects. *J Am Coll Nutr.* 2001;20.279 285.
57. Buddington RK, Williams CH, Chen SC, Witherly SA. Dietary supplement of neosugar alters the fecal flora and decreases activities of some reductive enzymes in human subjects. *Am J Clin Nutr.* 1996;63:709-716.
58. Klimberg VS, Salloum RM, Kasper M, et al. Oral glutamine accelerates healing of the small intestine and improves outcome after whole abdominal radiation. *Arch Surg.* 1990;125:1040-1045.
59. Souba WW, Klimberg VS, Plumley DA, et al. The role of glutamine in maintaining a healthy gut and supporting the metabolic response to injury and infection. *J Surg Res.* 1990;48:383-391.
60. Soeters PB, van de Poll MC, van Gemert WG, Dejong CH. Amino acid adequacy in pathophysiological states. *J Nutr.* 2004;134(Suppl 6):1575S-1582S.
61. Belluzzi A, Brignola C, Campieri M, et al. Effects of new fish oil derivative on fatty acid phospholipid-membrane pattern in a group of Crohn's disease patients. Dig Dis Sci. 1994;39:2589-2594.
62. Bjorkkjaer T, Brunborg LA, Arslan G, et al. Reduced joint pain after short-term duodenal administration of seal oil in patients with inflammatory bowel disease: comparison with soy oil. *Scand J Gastroenterol.* 2004;39:1088-1094.
63. Gil A. Polyunsaturated fatty acids and inflammatory diseases. *Biomed Pharmacother.* 2002;56:288-296.
64. Inui K, Fukuta Y, Ikeda A, Kameda H, Kokuba Y, Sato M. The nutritional effect of a-linolenic acid-rich emulsion with total parenteral nutrition in a rat model with inflammatory bowel disease. *Ann Nutr Metab.* 1996;40:227-233.
65. Lacroix B, Didier E, Grenier JF. Role of pantothenic and ascorbic acid in wound healing processes: in vitro study on fibroblasts. *Int J Vitam Nutr Res.* 1988;58:407-413.
66. Ellestad-Sayed JJ, Nelson RA, Adson MA, Palmer WM, Soule EH. Pantothenic acid, coenzyme A, and human chronic ulcerative and granulomatous colitis. *Am J Clin Nutr.* 1976;29:1333-1338.
67. Ojuawo A, Keith L. The serum concentrations of zinc, copper and selenium in children with inflammatory bowel disease. *Cent Afr J Med.* 2002;49(9-10):116-119.
68. Geerling BJ, Badart-Smook A, Stockbrugger RW, Brummer RJ. Comprehensive nutritional status in recently diagnosed patients with inflammatory bowel disease compared with population controls. *Eur J Clin Nutr.* 2000;54(6):514-521.
69. Fleming CR, Huizenga KA, McCall JT, Gildea J, Dennis R. Zinc nutrition in Crohn's disease. *Dig Dis Sci.* 1981;26(10):865-70.
70. Hendricks KM, Walker WA. Zinc deficiency in inflammatory bowel disease. *Nutr Rev.* 1988;46:401-408.

About the Authors

Leo Galland, MD, received the Linus Pauling Award from The Institute of Functional Medicine in 2000 for creating some of the basic principles underlying functional medicine. A board-certified internist, he has been applying nutritional therapies for the prevention and treatment of chronic disease for the past 30 years, and he is well known for his work on the relationship between intestinal health and systemic health. Dr. Galland received his education at Harvard University and the New York University School of Medicine, and he trained in internal medicine at Bellevue Hospital Center. He has held faculty positions at New York University, Rockefeller University, the Albert Einstein College of Medicine, the State University of New York at Stony Brook, and the University of Connecticut. Dr. Galland is a Fellow of the American College of Physicians and the American College of Nutrition and an Honorary Professor of the International College of Nutrition. He is the author of several dozen scientific articles and textbook chapters, as well as three books, *The Fat Resistance Diet*, *Power Healing*, and *Superimmunity for Kids*. In addition to his clinical practice in New York City, Dr. Galland is Director of The Foundation for Integrated Medicine (www.mdheal.org), a nonprofit educational organization, and the president of Applied Nutrition, Inc. (www.nutritionworkshop.com), which has created software for analyzing the interactions between drugs, diet, and dietary supplements.

Helen Lafferty, MB, MRCPI, was raised in Ireland, where she received her medical degree from University College Dublin in 1980. Following an internship, residency, and several years of medical practice in Ireland, she came to the United States, where she completed a clinical fellowship in nephrology in Providence, Rhode Island, and undertook several years of laboratory research in the Brigham and Women's Hospital/Harvard Medical School in Boston, Massachusetts. Following a career break to raise her three children, Dr. Lafferty is currently employed as a freelance medical writer and editor.